Springer Japan KK

K. Okita (Ed.)

Stem Cell and Liver Regeneration

With 28 Figures, Including 3 in Color

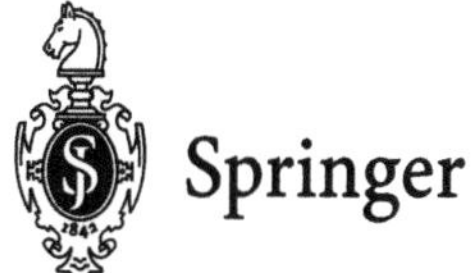

Springer

Kiwamu Okita, M.D., Ph.D.
Professor and Chairman
Department of Gastroenterology and Hepatology
Yamaguchi University School of Medicine
1-1-1 Minami-Kogushi, Ube, Yamaguchi 755-8505, Japan

Library of Congress Cataloging-in-Publication Data
Yamaguchi Symposium on Liver Disease (14th : 2002)
    Stem cell and liver regeneration / K. Okita, ed.
      p. ; cm.
    Includes bibliographical references and index.
    ISBN 978-4-431-67972-1   ISBN 978-4-431-53971-1 (eBook)
    DOI 10.1007/978-4-431-53971-1
        1. Liver—Diseases—Congresses. 2. Liver—Regeneration—Congresses. 3. Transplantation
of organs, tissues, etc.—Congresses. I. Okita, Kiwamu. II. Title.
    [DNLM: 1. Liver Diseases—therapy—Congresses. 2. Liver
Regeneration—genetics—Congresses. 3. Gene Therapy—methods—Congresses. 4. Stem Cell
Transplantation—Congresses. 5. Stem Cells—physiology—Congresses. WI700 Y19s 2004]
    RC846.Y364   2004
    616.3'62—dc22
                                                                                    2003057106

This symposium was supported by funds from the Viral Hepatitis Research Foundation of Japan.

Printed on acid-free paper

SPIN: 10932513

Preface

The considerable excitement surrounding the field of stem cells is based on the unique biological properties of these cells and their capacity to self-renew and regenerate tissue and organ systems. Although the existence of a liver stem cell has been debated for many years, it is now generally accepted that the liver contains cells with stem-like properties and that these cells can be activated to proliferate and differentiate into mature hepatocytes under certain pathophysiologic circumstances. Hepatic stem cells had been thought to be located in the canal of Hering in the liver, but recent work has demonstrated the existence of hepatic stem cells in bone marrow as well. Also in some experimental models, which induce liver damage and simultaneously block hepatocyte proliferation, the recruitment of a hepatic progenitor cell population consisting of oval cells is invariably observed. There is a substantial body of evidence to suggest that oval cells are involved in liver regeneration, as they differentiate into hepatocytes and biliary cells. However, the relation among hepatic stem cells, hepatic oval cells, and bone marrow cells is still obscure.

Cellular therapy with liver stem cells and their progeny including bone marrow cells is a promising new approach which will contribute to gene therapy of liver diseases. This book contains the most recent aspects of hepatic stem cell and liver regeneration and will contribute to future research in this field.

We thank the Otsuka Pharmaceutical Co. Ltd., for their continuing support.

Additionally, the Organizing Committee of the Yamaguchi Symposium and all participants are very grateful for the contribution of Professor Kenichi Kobayashi, a member of the Organizing Committee, who, sadly, passed away in 2002.

Organizing Committee of the Yamaguchi Symposium on Liver Disease

Kiwamu Okita, M.D., Yamaguchi University, Ube
Masamichi Kojiro, M.D., Kurume University, Kurume
Masao Omata, M.D., The University of Tokyo, Tokyo
Norio Hayashi, M.D., Osaka University, Osaka

Secretary General

Isao Sakaida, M.D., Yamaguchi University, Ube

Table of Contents

List of Participants

Chang, Mei-Hwei — Department of Pediatrics, College of Medicine
National Taiwan University, Taiwan, ROC

Chayama, Kazuki — First Department of Internal Medicine
Hiroshima University School of Medicine
Hiroshima, Japan

Hayashi, Norio — Department of Molecular Therapeutics
Osaka University Graduate School of Medicine
Osaka, Japan

Hino, Keisuke — Faculty of Health Sciences, Yamaguchi University
School of Medicine, Yamaguchi, Japan

Hino, Okio — Department of Experimental Pathology
Japanese Foundation for Cancer Research
Tokyo, Japan

Ichida, Takafumi — Third Department of Internal Medicine
Niigata University School of Medicine
Niigata, Japan

Ido, Akio — Second Department of Internal Medicine
Miyazaki Medical College, Miyazaki, Japan

Kakinuma, Sei — Department of Gastroenterology and Hepatology
Tokyo Medical and Dental University, Tokyo, Japan

Kimura, Teruaki — Department of Gastroenterology and Hepatology
Yamaguchi University School of Medicine
Yamaguchi, Japan

Kodama, Takahiro — Department of Internal Medicine/Gastroenterology
Yamaguchi Central Hospital, Yamaguchi, Japan

Kojiro, Masamichi — Department of Pathology
Kurume University School of Medicine
Fukuoka, Japan

Kurokawa, Fumie

Department of Gastroenterology and Hepatology
Yamaguchi University School of Medicine
Yamaguchi, Japan

Nakamura, Koji

Stem Cell Regulation Project
Kanagawa Academy of Science and Technology
(KAST), Kanagawa, Japan

Nakanishi, Toshio

Department of Radiology
Hiroshima University School of Medicine
Hiroshima, Japan

Nishina, Hiroshi

Department of Physiological Chemistry
Graduate School of Pharmaceutical Sciences
The University of Tokyo, Tokyo, Japan

Okita, Kiwamu

Department of Gastroenterology and Hepatology
Yamaguchi University School of Medicine
Yamaguchi, Japan

Sakaida, Isao

Department of Gastroenterology and Hepatology
Yamaguchi University School of Medicine
Yamaguchi, Japan

Shafritz, David A.

Marion Bessin Liver Research Center
Albert Einstein College of Medicine, New York, U.S.A.

Takehara, Tetsuo

Department of Molecular Therapeutics
Osaka University Graduate School of Medicine
Osaka, Japan

Tanaka, Yujiro

Department of General Medicine
Tokyo Medical and Dental University, Tokyo, Japan

Taniguchi, Eitaro

Second Department of Internal Medicine
Kurume University School of Medicine
Fukuoka, Japan

Tanikawa, Kyuichi

International Institute for Liver Research
Fukuoka, Japan

Terai, Shuji

Department of Gastroenterology and Hepatology
Yamaguchi University School of Medicine
Yamaguchi, Japan

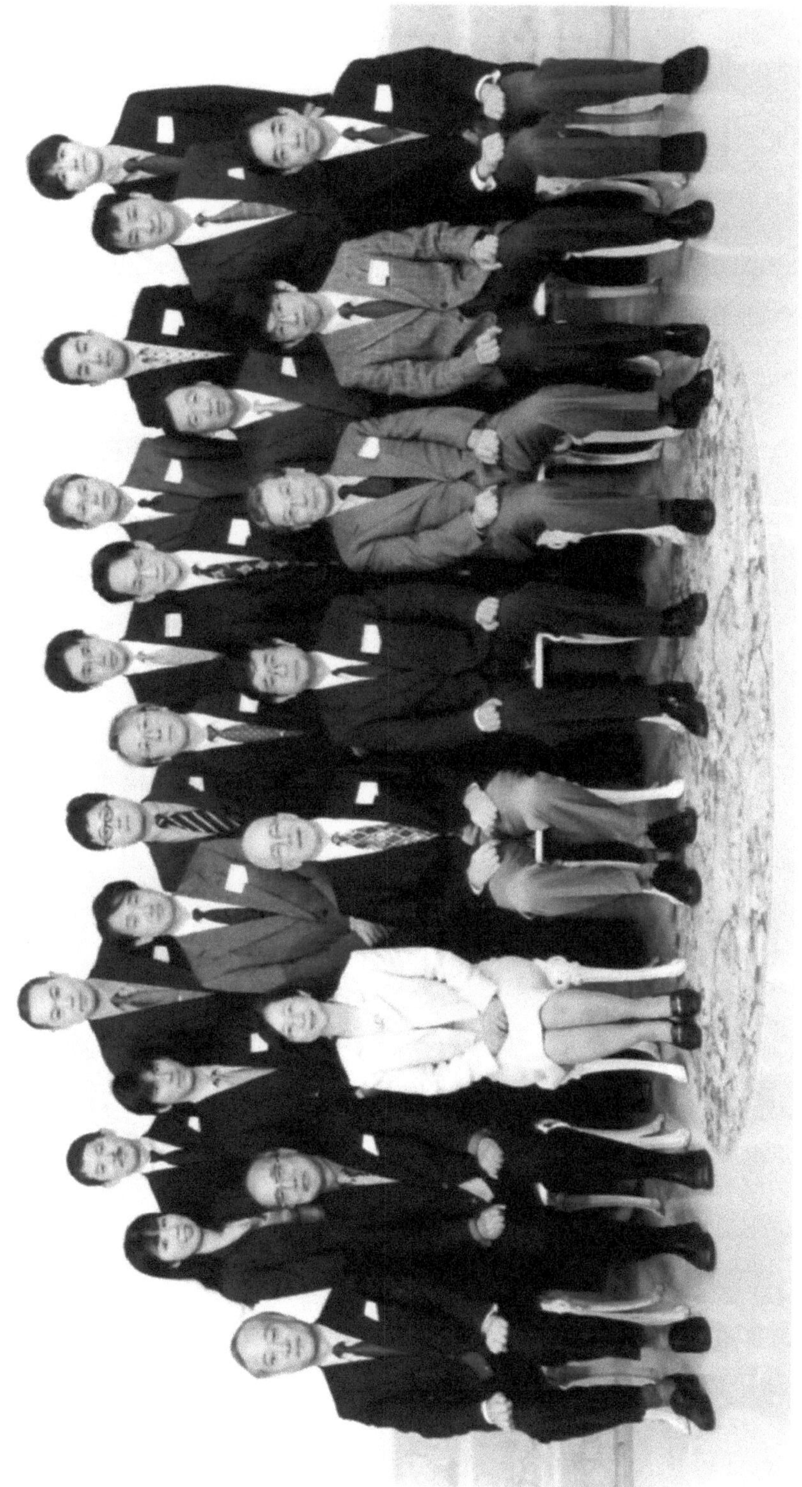

SAPK/JNK Signaling Participates in Embryonic Hepatoblast Proliferation via a Pathway Different from NF-κB-Induced Anti-Apoptosis

Hiroshi Nishina, Tomomi Watanabe, Kentaro Nakagawa, Shinya Ohata, Satoshi Asaka, and Toshiaki Katada

Summary. Mice lacking the stress-signaling kinases SEK1 and MKK7 die from embryonic day 10.5 (E10.5) to E12.5 with a defect in liver formation. However, the mechanism of the liver defect has remained unknown. In this review, we first introduce a monoclonal antibody, anti-Liv2, which specifically recognizes murine hepatoblasts, for the analysis of liver development, and further, we describe the genetic interaction of *sek1* with the tumor necrosis factor-α receptor 1 gene (*tnfr1*) and the protooncogene *c-jun*, which are also responsible for liver formation and cell apoptosis. The defective liver formation in *sek1*$^{-/-}$ embryos was not protected by an additional *tnfr1* mutation that rescues the embryonic lethality of mice lacking nuclear factor-kappa B (NF-κB) signaling components. There was a progressive increase in hepatoblast cell numbers in wild-type embryos from E10.5 to E12.5. In contrast, impaired hepatoblast proliferation was observed in *sek1*$^{-/-}$ livers from E10.5, although fetal liver-specific gene expression was normal. The impaired phenotype in *sek1*$^{-/-}$ livers was more severe than that in *c-jun*$^{-/-}$ embryos, and *sek1*$^{-/-}$ *c-jun*$^{-/-}$ embryos died earlier before E8.5. The hepatoblast proliferation required no hematopoiesis, because liver development was not impaired in *AML1*$^{-/-}$ mice, which lack hematopoietic functions. Stimulation of stress-activated protein kinase/c-Jun N-terminal kinase (SAPK/JNK) by hepatocyte growth factor was attenuated in *sek1*$^{-/-}$ livers. Thus, SEK1 and MKK7-mediated SAPK/JNK signaling appears to play a crucial role in hepatoblast proliferation and survival in a manner that is apparently different from that of NF-κB or c-Jun.

Key words. SEK1, NF-κB, SAPK/JNK, Hepatoblast, Hepatogenesis

Introduction

Embryonic liver formation consists of multiple stages and is under the influence of hormonal factors, as well as intercellular and matrix-cellular interactions. In mice, the initial event of liver ontogeny occurs around embryonic day 9 (E9), when epithelial cells of the foregut endoderm commit to become the liver primordium through their interaction with the cardiogenic mesoderm. The liver primordium proliferates and

Department of Physiological Chemistry, Graduate School of Pharmaceutical Sciences, The University of Tokyo, 7-3-1 Hongo, Bunkyo-ku, Tokyo 113-0033, Japan

invades the mesenchyme of the septum transversum to give rise to the hepatic codes and bud at E9.5. A critical genetic checkpoint in embryogenesis is the switch from yolk sac- and aorta-gonad-mesonephros region-dependent blood formation to liver-dependent hematopoiesis. This switch in the hematopoietic organ occurs from E10.5 to E12.5. The next major stage occurs around E14.5 when both hepatocytes and bile-duct epithelial cells arise embryologically from a common founder cell, the hepato-blast, which has bipotential differentiation capabilities in liver development [1,2].

The degree of hepatic maturation has been characterized by the expression of liver- and stage-specific genes [3,4]. Alphafetoprotein (AFP) is an early fetal hepatic marker (E9), and its expression decreases as the liver develops [5]. In contrast, the expression of albumin, the most abundant protein synthesized by hepatocytes, starts in early fetal hepatocytes (E12) and reaches the maximal level in the adult [6]. However, antibod-ies specific for AFP or albumin are not adequate to estimate the precise numbers of hepatoblasts in early fetal livers at E9.5–12.5, because both are diffusible serum pro-teins. Therefore, novel antibodies that clearly and specifically recognize individual hepatoblasts are required for studying fetal liver development in detail [7].

Recently, it has been shown by using ventral foregut endoderm isolated from mouse embryos at E8.25, that the close proximity of the cardiac mesoderm, which expresses fibroblast growth factors (FGFs) 1, 2, and 8, causes the foregut endoderm to develop into the liver [8,9]. On the other hand, another recent report has indicated a paracrine mechanism of late hepatogenesis that is derived from E14.5 murine embryos in cul-tured fetal liver cells. Blood cells in the fetal liver produce an interleukin (IL) 6-family cytokine, oncostatin M (OSM), to promote the development of hepatocytes [10]. However, the relationship between hepatogenesis and hematopoiesis in early fetal liver development remains unclear.

The stress-activated protein kinase/extracellular signal-regulated kinase kinases, SEK1/MKK4 and SEK2/MKK7, are direct activators of the stress-activated protein kinase (SAPK; also called c-Jun N-terminal kinase; JNK). Both are activated in response to a variety of cellular stresses, such as changes in osmolarity, metabolic poisons, DNA damage, heat shock, or the inflammatory cytokines, IL-1 and tumor necrosis factor-α (TNF-α). SEK1 and/or MKK7-mediated activation of SAPK/JNK phosphorylates c-Jun and activates c-Jun/Fos heterodimeric (AP-1) transcriptional complexes [11,12]. Several groups, including ours, have disrupted the *sek1* gene in mice, using homolo-gous recombination [13–17]. SEK1-deficient embryos displayed severe anemia and died between E10.5 and E12.5. Hematopoiesis from yolk-sac precursors and vasculo-genesis were normal in SEK1-deficient embryos. However, hepatogenesis and liver for-mation were severely impaired in the mutant embryos, and SEK1-deficient embryos had greatly reduced numbers of hepatocytes at E11.5–12.5. Although formation of the primordial liver and hepatic bud appeared to be normal, SEK1-deficient hepatocytes underwent massive apoptosis at E12.5 [15,17]. Embryos lacking the *c-jun* gene also display defective liver organization and die between E11.5 and E15.5 [18,19]. These results indicate that SEK1 and c-Jun provide a crucial and specific survival signal for fetal hepatogenesis. It is as yet unclear where SEK1 plays a role in hematopoietic cells or in hepatogenesis, what receptors trigger SEK1 activation, and what molecules regu-late the SEK1-mediated signaling pathway in fetal liver development.

TNF-α elicits a wide range of biological responses, such as inflammation, tumor necrosis, differentiation, cell proliferation, and apoptosis, through the stimulation of its receptor, TNFR1. Recently, it has been revealed that three separate signaling pathways, the induction of apoptosis, nuclear factor-kappa B (NF-κB) activation, and SEK1 and/or MKK7-mediated SAPK/JNK activation, are simultaneously mediated through TNFR1, and that SAPK/JNK activation appears to be not involved in the TNFR1-dependent induction of apoptosis, while the activation of NF-κB protects against the apoptosis [20]. Knockout mice for genes that are involved in NF-κB signaling have massive liver degeneration and apoptosis during midgestation, at E12.5–16. Such mice include knockout mice, for the RelA subunit of transcription factor NF-κB (died at E15–16), IκB kinase (β/IKK2; died at E12.5–14), NEMO/IKKγ (died at E12.5–13.0), and TRAF2-associated kinase T2K; died at E12.5–14.5) [21–26]. Importantly, the embryonic lethality and liver apoptosis observed in RelA-, IKK2- and T2K-knockout mice can be rescued by the simultaneous inactivation of TNFR1, suggesting that the apoptosis is induced by TNF-α circulating in the embryos [22,26,27]. However, the physiological role of the SEK1 and/or MKK7-mediated activation of SAPK/JNK in response to TNFR1 ligation remains to be resolved [20].

To understand the mechanisms of defective liver formation, we prepared monoclonal antibodies that specifically recognized murine fetal livers and characterized them using paraffin sections of embryos at various stages. One of the antibodies called anti-Liv2, specifically recognized so-called hepatoblasts at E9.5–12.5. We examined the relationship between the lethality of $sek1^{-/-}$ embryos and TNFR1-mediated apoptosis in mice lacking these genes. We found that $sek1^{-/-}$ $tnfr1^{-/-}$ double-mutant embryos delayed the beginning of liver resorption by 2 days compared with $sek1^{-/-}$ $tnfr1^{+/-}$ embryos, and that the liver defect was not rescued by the $sek1^{-/-}$ $tnfr1^{-/-}$ genotype. In addition, we investigated the ability of hepatoblast growth, as judged by the incorporation of bromodeoxyuridine (BrdU), in $sek1^{-/-}$ embryos at E10.5 before the occurrence of defective liver formation and massive apoptosis. We found a growth defect of hepatoblasts in $sek1^{-/-}$ embryos at E10.5. Furthermore, we showed that hepatoblasts could develop without hematopoiesis in early fetal liver at E9.5–11.5, using $AML1^{-/-}$ embryos, which lack definitive hematopoiesis [28,29]. The activation of SAPK/JNK by hepatocyte growth factor (HGF), observable in wild-type fetal livers, was markedly impaired in $sek1^{-/-}$ fetal livers. Thus, the lethality of $sek1$ mutant embryos is most likely due to a defect that reflects SEK1 function and is not associated with NF-κB-induced anti-apoptosis in the cell growth of hepatoblasts [7].

A Novel Monoclonal Antibody, Anti-Liv2, Specifically Recognizes Hepatoblasts in Murine Embryos

To investigate fetal liver development in murine embryos at the early stage of E9.5–12.5, we prepared novel rat monoclonal antibodies against the fetal livers at E11.5 [7]. As shown in Fig. 1, one of the antibodies, anti-Liv2, specifically recognized hepatic cells that were co-stained with anti-HNF-3β antibody (Fig. 1A,B,D), but did not recognize TER119-positive erythrocytes. Although the nature of the Liv2 antigen has not been identified yet, the cell membrane of hepatic cells was stained with the monoclonal antibody, but the cytoplasm and nuclei were not (Fig. 1C). Almost all cells in the hepatic bud at E9.5 were recognized by anti-Liv2 (Fig. 1E,F). Interestingly, there was a progressive decrease in the ratio of Liv2-positive cells to the total number of

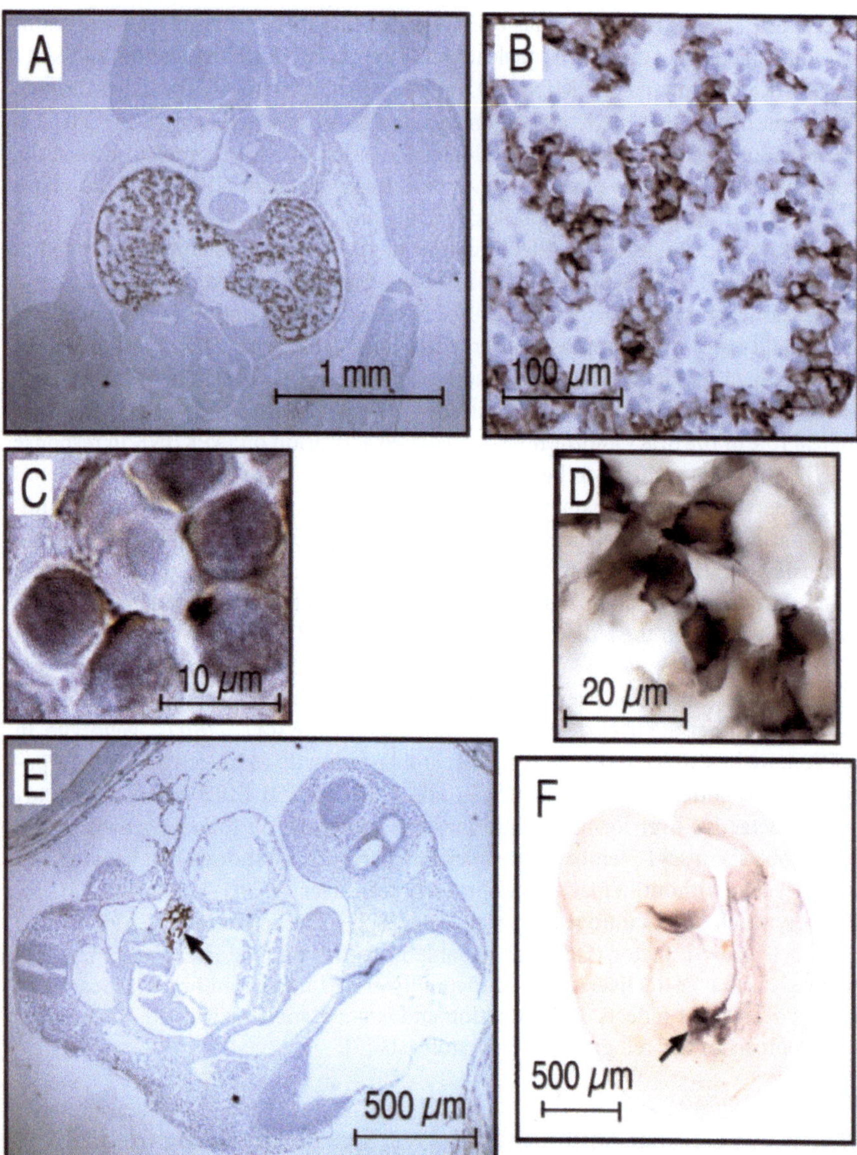

Fig. 1A–F. Characterization of a novel rat monoclonal antibody, anti-Liv2, which shows specific recognition of hepatoblasts in murine embryos. Transverse paraffin sections of murine embryonic livers at embryonic day 11.5 (E11.5) (**A–C**) and E9.5 (**E**), together with a frozen section at E11.5 (**D**) and a whole embryo at E9.5 (**F**), were stained with the rat monoclonal antibody, anti-Liv2. Positive cells exhibit a *brown* (**A–C**, and **E**) or *dark blue* (**D** and **E**) precipitate. **D** The frozen section containing Liv2-positive cells (*dark blue*) was further stained with anti-HNF-3β (*brown*). The *arrows* show hepatic buds

cells as the fetal liver developed from E9.5 to E12.5. Thus, it is very likely that anti-Liv2 specifically recognizes the so-called hepatoblasts that appear with fetal liver development. This monoclonal antibody was employed in the present study as a useful tool to analyze hepatoblasts in various mutant mice.

A Different Role of SEK1 from that of NF-κB-Induced Anti-Apoptosis in Fetal Liver Formation

As mentioned in the "Introduction", mice lacking SEK1 or NF-κB signaling components show embryonic lethality, with impaired liver formation, furthermore, the activation of both SEK1 and NF-κB is induced by TNFR1 in the fetal livers. Interestingly, liver apoptosis originating from the lack of NF-κB signaling components was rescued by the inactivation of TNFR1 [22,26,27]. Therefore, we investigated the relationship between SEK1- and TNFR1-mediated signaling pathways in whole embryos and fetal livers. C57BL/6-background $sek1^{-/-}$ $tnfr1^{-/-}$ embryos were prepared from $sek1^{+/-}$ $tnfr1^{-/-}$ intercrosses, and $sek1^{-/-}$ $tnfr1^{+/-}$ embryos were prepared from $sek1^{+/-}$ $tnfr1^{-/-}$ and $sek1^{+/-}$ $tnfr1^{+/+}$ intercrosses (Table 1). Embryos of all three expected genotypes from $sek1^{+/-}$ $tnfr1^{-/-}$ and $sek1^{+/-}$ $tnfr1^{+/+}$ intercrosses were not present at normal Mendelian ratios at E12.5 (Table 1, left side). Interestingly, embryos of all three expected genotypes from $sek1^{+/-}$ $tnfr1^{-/-}$ intercrosses were present at the normal Mendelian ratios until E13.5 and became abnormal at E14.5 (Table 1, right side). Embryo resorption was thus rescued by 2 days. The apparent sizes of $sek1^{-/-}$ $tnfr1^{-/-}$ embryos and livers were almost the same as those of the wild-type at E11.5 (Fig. 2A,B). However, liver defects were not rescued in $sek1^{-/-}$ $tnfr1^{-/-}$ embryos (Fig. 2E,G). The SEK1-deficient livers contained a capsule, hematopoietic precursors, and disorganized islands of Liv2-positive hepatoblasts (Fig. 2F), and these defects were still observed in $sek1^{-/-}$ $tnfr1^{-/-}$ livers (Fig. 2E,G). These results clearly indicate that embryo resorption is partially due to TNFR1-mediated signaling and that the role of SEK1 in fetal liver formation is different from that of NF-κB signaling, whose defects were rescued by inactivation of TNFR1 function.

Table 1. Analysis of embryos obtained from $sek1^{+/-}$ $tnfr1^{-/-}$ intercrosses or $sek1^{+/-}$ $tnfr1^{-/-}$ and $sek1^{+/-}$ $tnfr1^{+/+}$ intercrosses

Embryonic stage	$sek1^{+/+}$ $tnfr1^{+/-}$	$sek1^{+/-}$ $tnfr1^{+/-}$	$sek1^{-/-}$ $tnfr1^{+/-}$	$sek1^{+/+}$ $tnfr1^{-/-}$	$sek1^{+/-}$ $tnfr1^{-/-}$	$sek1^{-/-}$ $tnfr1^{-/-}$
E12.5	4	6	1*	12	34	15
E13.5	11	23	6*	17	33	17
E14.5	ND	ND	ND	9	16	1*

Asterisks indicate that embryos were under conditions of resorption
Embryos were isolated at the indicated time points of gestation and analyzed for Mendelian ratios of all three expected genotypes. Genotypes of embryos were determined by polymerase chain reaction (PCR), and the numbers of each genotype are listed in the Table.
ND, not determined

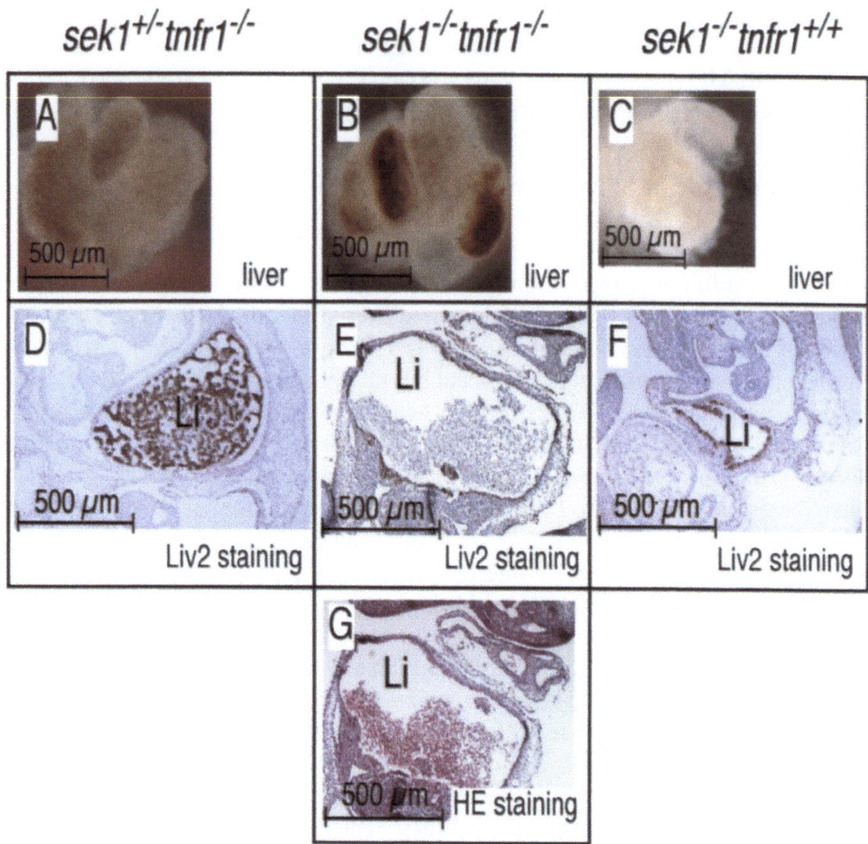

Fig. 2A–G. No rescue by tumor necrosis factory-α receptor 1 (TNFR1) inactivation of defective liver formation in *sek1$^{-/-}$* embryos. Microscopic analysis was performed in *sek$^{+/-}$ tnfr1$^{-/-}$* (**A** and **D**), *sek1$^{-/-}$ tnfr1$^{-/-}$* (**B, E,** and **G**), and *sek1$^{-/-}$ tnfr1$^{+/+}$* (**C** and **F**) fetal livers at E11.5. Transverse sections were stained with anti-Liv2 (**D–F**) and HE (**G**). *Li*, liver. *Bars*, 500 μm

SEK1-Deficient Livers Show a Decreased Number of Hepatoblasts in Early Hepatogenesis

To characterize *sek1$^{-/-}$* livers, we determined numbers of Liv2-positive cells in *c-jun$^{-/-}$* embryos, which also have defective liver formation [18,30]. Total cell numbers in *sek1$^{-/-}$* and *c-jun$^{-/-}$* livers were significantly lower than those in the wild-type liver. However, the ratio of Liv2-positive to the total number of liver cells was not significantly different among the three types of mice, and the ratios gradually decreased with liver development, being approximately 100% at E9.5, 60% at E10.5, 50% at E11.5, and 20% at E12.5. The number of Liv2-positive cells increased progressively, from 5×10^4 to 3×10^5 cells, during E10.5–12.5 in wild-type fetal livers. Although the numbers of Liv2-positive cells at E10.5 were not different among wild-type, *sek1$^{-/-}$*, and *c-jun$^{-/-}$* livers, the progressive increase observed in wild-type livers was markedly attenuated at E11.5 and E12.5 in *sek1*$^{-/-}$ and *c-jun*$^{-/-}$ livers, respectively. These results clearly indicate that impaired hepatoblast development certainly occurs in *sek1*$^{-/-}$ embryos and that *sek1* mutation is more severe than *c-jun* mutation in terms of hepatoblast development, which is consistent with the previous finding that *sek1*$^{-/-}$ embryos die earlier than *c-jun*$^{-/-}$ embryos.

SEK1-Deficient Livers Exhibit Normal Hepatic Gene Expression

A recent study has shown that *c-jun*$^{-/-}$ livers display the normal expression of the mRNAs, for albumin, keratin 18, hepatocyte HNF-1, β-globin, and erythropoietin, some of which are putative AP-1 target genes [30]. To confirm normal liver differentiation in *sek1*$^{-/-}$ embryos, the tissue-specific gene expression was measured by means of reverse transcription-polymerase chain reaction (RT-PCR). An early fetal hepatic marker, AFP, was expressed at the same level in wild-type and *sek1*$^{-/-}$ livers at E10.5 when cell numbers of Liv2-positive hepatoblasts were the same. Furthermore, a mature hepatic marker, albumin, was also expressed in both wild-type and *sek1*$^{-/-}$ fetal livers at E10.5 and E11.5. These results indicate that hepatic differentiation is not affected in *sek1*$^{-/-}$ fetal livers, similar to findings in *c-jun*$^{-/-}$ livers.

SEK1-Deficient Livers are Characterized as Showing Impaired Cell Growth of Hepatoblasts

We previously reported massive cell apoptosis in *sek1*$^{-/-}$ livers at E12.5 [15]. This apoptosis appeared to be associated with a decreased number of hepatoblasts at E11.5, without significant change in the gene expression of hepatic markers. Therefore, the growth capacity of *sek1*$^{-/-}$ hepatoblasts at the early stage of E10.5 was analyzed by the incorporation of bromodeoxyuridine (BrdU; Fig. 3). Interestingly, BrdU incorporation into Liv2-positive hepatoblasts was greatly reduced in *sek1*$^{-/-}$ livers compared with wild-type and *c-jun*$^{-/-}$ livers. These results suggest that *sek1* mutation may result in the impaired growth capacity of hepatoblasts at E10.5 when no other obvious defects in *sek1*$^{-/-}$ livers are observed.

Genetic Interaction Between *sek1* and *c-jun* in Murine Development

Because *sek1* and *c-jun* knockout mice display a similar phenotype of impaired liver formation [15], we further examined the genetic interaction between the two genes by preparing *sek1*$^{-/-}$ *c-jun*$^{-/-}$ double-mutant embryos. According to the Mendelian ratio (1:16), there was the expected number of the *sek1*$^{-/-}$ *c-jun*$^{-/-}$ genotype in E8.5 embryos, in addition to *sek1*$^{+/+}$ *c-jun*$^{+/+}$, *sek1*$^{-/-}$ *c-jun*$^{+/+}$, and *sek1*$^{+/+}$ *c-jun*$^{-/-}$ genotypes. No *sek1*$^{-/-}$ *c-jun*$^{-/-}$ embryos were, however, observed at E10.5, though embryos of the *sek1* or *c-jun* single mutant existed at the expected numbers. The loss of *sek1*$^{-/-}$ *c-jun*$^{-/-}$ embryos at E10.5 appeared to be due to resorption, because all the embryos at E8.5 were already dead. Thus, *sek1*$^{-/-}$ *c-jun*$^{-/-}$ double-mutant embryos died before E8.5 and underwent resorption through E10.5. These results indicate that the *sek1* and *c-jun* genes work synergistically during early embryonic development.

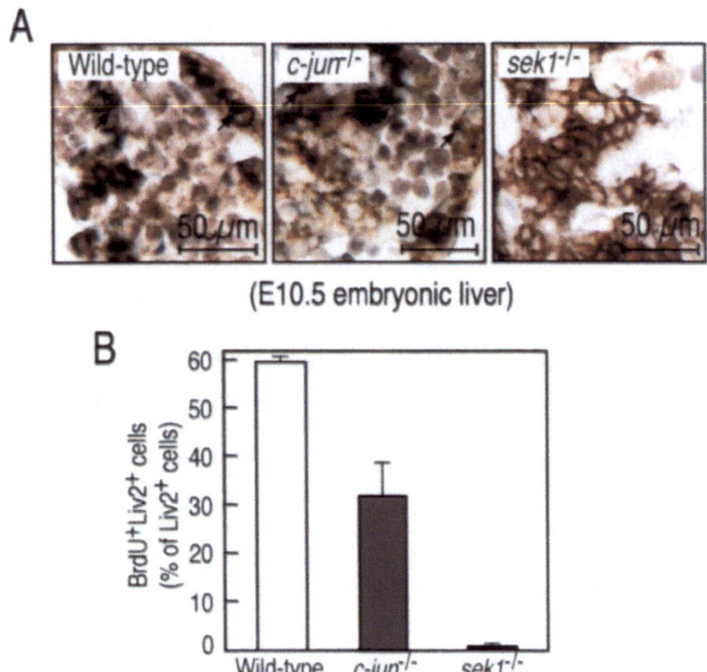

Fig. 3A,B. Impaired hepatoblast growth observed in *sek1*$^{-/-}$ livers. Pregnant mice bearing E10.5 embryos were injected with 0.3 ml of 50 mg/ml bromo-deoxyuridine (*BrdU*). After 4 h, the embryos were isolated, fixed with 4% paraformaldehyde, and genotypes of the embryos were determined by polymerase chain reaction (PCR). **A** Transverse sections were prepared from the paraffin embedding of wild-type (*left*), *c-jun*$^{-/-}$ (*middle*), and *sek1*$^{-/-}$ (*right*) embryos and stained with anti-Liv2 (*brown*). *Arrows* indicate BrdU-incorporated (*blue colored*) Liv2-positive hepatoblasts. **B** The BrdU-incorporated cells were counted in the three embryos (wild-type, *c-jun*$^{-/-}$, and *sek1*$^{-/-}$), and the values are expressed as percentages of the total of Liv2-positive hepatoblasts

No Requirement of Hematopoiesis for Hepatoblast Growth in Early Hepatogenesis

To examine the relationship between hepatoblast growth and hematopoiesis in early fetal liver, we measured the number of Liv2-positive cells at E11.5 in *AML1*$^{-/-}$ embryos, which lack definitive hematopoiesis. The total numbers of hepatic cells *plus* blood cells in wild-type and *AML1*$^{-/-}$ livers at E11.5 were counted, at 3.0×10^5 and 2.2×10^5 cells, respectively. When paraffin sections were prepared from E11.5 fetal livers and stained with anti-Liv2 or anti-TER119, there were 44% and 79% of Liv2-positive cells in wild-type and *AML1*$^{-/-}$ livers, respectively. *AML1*$^{-/-}$ fetal livers at E11.5 contained approximately 80% of Liv2-positive cells and 20% of TER119-positive primitive erythrocytes. Therefore, the numbers of Liv2-positive cells were calculated to be 1.3×10^5 and 1.7×10^5 in wild-type and *AML1*$^{-/-}$ livers, respectively. Thus, the cell numbers of hepatoblasts were higher in *AML1*$^{-/-}$ livers than in wild-type ones. These results indicate that hematopoiesis and growth factors from blood cells are not essentially required for hepatoblast growth in early hepatogenesis.

Impairment of HGF-Induced SAPK/JNK Activation in Fetal Livers Lacking SEK1

To elucidate the biochemical interaction between SEK1 and SAPK/JNK, we first investigated whether HGF, which is produced by nonblood cells, could activate SAPK/JNK in fetal liver cells expressing the HGF receptor, c-Met. In a previous report [15], we could not detect any SAPK/JNK activation by HGF in a primary cell culture prepared from fetal livers. Therefore, in this study, we screened liver cells in an intact condition and found that strong SAPK/JNK activation was observed in response to HGF by using whole livers at E10.5, where about 60% of cells are Liv2-positive hepatoblasts. There was maximally a more than 25-fold increase in SAPK/JNK activity at 10 min, and the activity decreased rapidly. Such marked activation of SAPK/JNK was, however, greatly reduced in *sek1*$^{-/-}$ fetal livers. Interestingly, another member of the stress-activated mitogen activated protein (MAP) kinase family, p38, was constitutively phosphorylated without stimulation by HGF in fetal livers, and this phosphorylation was still observed in *sek1*$^{-/-}$ fetal livers. These results indicate that SEK1 is required for HGF-induced full activation of SAPK/JNK but not for p38 activation, and that HGF is one of the growth factors that regulate hepatoblast growth in early fetal liver development.

Conclusion

Embryonic liver formation is, genetically, a crucial checkpoint in fetal hematopoiesis and development. Although hematopoiesis has been characterized at the cellular and molecular levels, hepatogenesis and liver formation are just beginning to be characterized. To analyze early liver development, we first screened monoclonal antibodies that specifically recognized murine fetal livers by using transverse sections of E11.5 embryos. One of the antibodies, anti-Liv2, is applicable to paraffin sections and whole mount embryos, and the Liv2 antigen appears to be localized in the cell membrane (Fig. 1). The ratios of Liv2-positive cells from E9.5 to E12.5 were consistent with those of hepatic cells defined as hepatoblasts. Using anti-Liv2, we measured the exact cell numbers of hepatoblasts in fetal liver development in wild-type, *sek1*$^{-/-}$, and *c-jun*$^{-/-}$ mice. Thus, our experiments proved anti-Liv2 to be a useful tool for identifying murine hepatoblasts in early fetal livers, though the Liv2 antigen and its physiological role have not been determined yet.

Previously, we and another group reported that *sek1*$^{-/-}$ embryos died between E10.5 and E12.5, with a decreased number of cytokeratin-positive hepatocytes at E11.5, and massive hepatocyte apoptosis at E12.5 [15,17]. To extend the above results, we examined an interesting question: whether the hepatic apoptosis and embryonic lethality observed in *sek1*$^{-/-}$ mice are rescued by the introduction of *tnfr1* gene mutation (Table 1 and Fig. 2). As shown in Fig. 4, TNFR1 relays TNF-α stimulation to three separate pathways, which include the induction of apoptosis, NF-κB activation, and SAPK/JNK activation [20]. Activation of NF-κB protects against TNF-α-induced apoptosis.

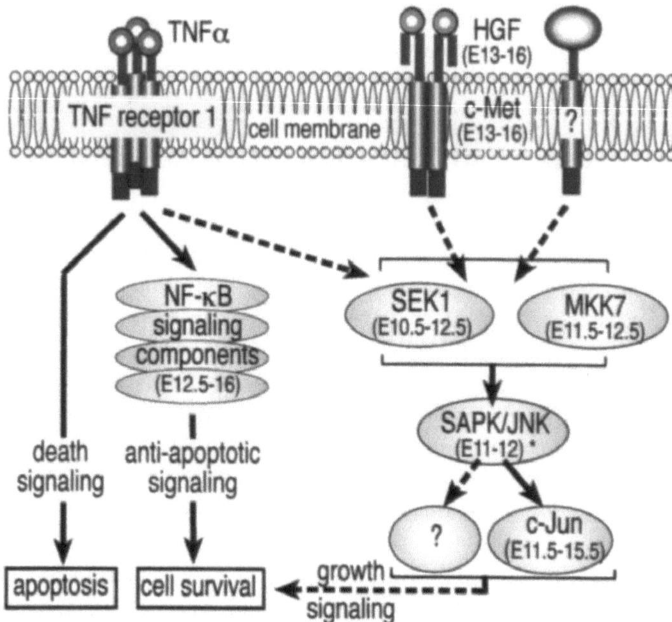

Fig. 4. Proposed model for SEK1-associated signaling pathways in hepatoblasts. The *numbers in parentheses* are days of embryonic lethality reported in previous studies and in the present study. *Solid* and *broken lines* show signaling pathways reported in previous studies and the present study, respectively. *Asterisk* indicates that $Jnk1^{-/-}$ $Jnk2^{-/-}$ mutant mice die between the eleventh and twelfth days of gestation [42] *TNF* α, tumor necrosis factor alpha, *HGF*, hepatocyte growth factor; *NF-κB*, nuclear factor kappa B; *SAPK/JNK*, stress-activated protein kinase/c-Jun N-terminal kinase

Therefore, mice lacking components of the NF-κB signaling pathway, such as RelA, IKK2, NEMO, or T2K show embryonic lethality, with massive liver apoptosis, and are rescued by the introduction of *tnfr1* mutaion. However, the physiological role of SEK1 and/or MKK7-mediated SAPK/JNK activation in response to TNFR1 stimulation remains to be resolved. In the present study, we examined the phenotype of body sizes and fetal livers of both SEK1 and TNFR1 double-knockout mice. Interestingly, embryo resorption was partially inhibited in $sek1^{-/-}$ $tnfr1^{-/-}$ mice, although the liver defect induced by *sek1* mutation was not rescued (Table 1 and Fig. 2). These results clearly show that the SEK1-mediated signal plays an important role, which is apparently different from the NF-κB signal, in fetal liver formation. Another important conclusion from the results with the $sek1^{-/-}$ $tnfr1^{-/-}$ mice is that TNFR1 plays a role in embryo resorption. Some studies have suggested the involvement of TNF-α in embryo loss and resorption by showing changes in its expression [31–33]. Our genetic experiments showing partial rescue of embryo resorption by the inactivation of TNFR1 function are consistent with the idea that TNFR1-mediated death signaling plays a role in the clearance of abnormal embryos. Thus, TNF-α elicits a wide spectrum of cellular responses, including apoptosis and cell growth. TNFR1 may relay its stimulation to SEK1-mediated cell growth in hepatoblasts, resulting in cell survival. The balance of three separate pathways may be important for eliciting various cellular responses, depending on the type of cell and its developmental stage (Fig. 4).

To find the primary cause of the liver defect caused by *sek1* mutation, we analyzed *sek1*$^{-/-}$ livers using anti-Liv2 and found decreased numbers of hepatoblasts in the mutant embryos at E11.5. Furthermore, we found impaired BrdU incorporation into Liv2-positive hepatoblasts in *sek1*$^{-/-}$ livers at E10.5 (Fig. 3). Because liver-specific gene expression was normal in *sek1*$^{-/-}$ fetal livers, the liver defects in *sek1*$^{-/-}$ embryos are very likely due to the impaired cell growth of hepatoblasts in early hepatogenesis, resulting in decreased numbers of hepatoblasts and massive hepatoblast apoptosis. A recent report showing the maturation of SEK1-null embryonic stem cells into a hepatic lineage in vitro also indicates that the liver defect caused by *sek1* mutation is not due to impaired differentiation or maturation of hepatocytes [34]. Thus, SEK1 may provide crucial and specific growth and survival signals for hepatoblasts.

Interestingly, the findings of impaired SAPK/JNK activation in *sek1*$^{-/-}$ fetal livers extend our recent report that the synergistic activation of SAPK/JNK is impaired in SEK1-deficient murine embryonic stem cells and MKK7-deficient murine mast cells [35,36]. Furthermore, mice lacking MKK7 also show embryonic lethality between E11.5 and E12.5, with impaired liver formation and a decreased level of SAPK/JNK activation (our unpublished data). Thus, the synergistic activation of SAPK/JNK by SEK1 and MKK7 seems to occur in fetal livers and seems to be crucial for hepatoblast growth in mouse development (Fig. 4).

As described above, hepatoblast development in early hepatogenesis does not require definitive hematopoiesis. Therefore, growth factor(s), produced by nonblood cells, together with their receptor(s) on hepatoblasts, could relay SEK1 activation and promote cell growth and cell survival (Fig. 4). This idea is supported by a recent report showing that vasculogenic endothelial cells and nascent vessels are critical for the earliest stages of hepatogenesis, prior to blood-vessel function [37]. Various growth factors, such as HGF, epidermal growth factor, IL-1, and TNF-α have been implicated in hepatogenesis [38]. However, mice lacking the *TNF-α, TNFR1, IL-1,* or *IL-1R* genes did not have any defects in liver formation [39]. By contrast, HGF-deficient mice die between E13 and E16 with liver failure, and the embryonic livers are reduced in size and show extensive loss of hepatocytes [40,41]. We found that HGF is capable of stimulating SAPK/JNK activity in wild-type fetal livers at E10.5 and that the activation is markedly impaired in *sek1*$^{-/-}$ fetal livers. Thus, the HGF receptor, c-Met, is one of the candidates for relaying SEK1 activation and promoting hepatoblast growth and survival. However, *hgf*$^{-/-}$ mice die later than *sek1*$^{-/-}$ mice and have an additional defect in placental development [40,41]. Therefore, another factor(s), which could also induce SEK1 activation, may be more essential for hepatoblast growth in early hepatogenesis (Fig. 4). Thus, SEK1 may receive various signals from cell-surface receptors to regulate hepatoblast growth and survival in murine embryogenesis.

References

1. LeDouarin NM (1975) An experimental analysis of liver development. Med Biol 53: 427–455
2. Houssaint E (1980) Differentiation of the mouse hepatic primordium. I. An analysis of tissue interactions in hepatocyte differentiation. Cell Differ 9:269–279

3. Derman E, Krauter K, Walling L, Weinberger C, Ray M, Darnell JE Jr (1981) Transcriptional control in the production of liver-specific mRNAs. Cell 23:731–739

4. Panduro A, Shalaby F, Shafritz DA (1987) Changing patterns of transcriptional and post-transcriptional control of liver-specific gene expression during rat development. Genes Dev 1:1172–1182

5. Shiojiri N, Lemire JM, Fausto N (1991) Cell lineages and oval cell progenitors in rat liver development. Cancer Res 51:2611–2620

6. Tilghman SM, Belayew A (1982) Transcriptional control of the murine albumin/alpha-fetoprotein locus during development. Proc Natl Acad Sci USA 79:5254–5257

7. Watanabe T, Nakagawa K, Ohata S, Kitagawa D, Nishitai G, Seo J, Tanemura S, Shimizu N, Kishimoto H, Wada T, Aoki J, Arai H, Iwatsubo T, Mochita M, Watanabe T, Satake M, Ito Y, Matsuyama T, Mak TW, Penninger JM, Nishina H, Katada T (2002) SEK1/MKK4-mediated SAPK/JNK signaling participates in embryonic hepatoblast proliferation via a pathway different from NF-κB-induced anti-apoptosis. Dev Biol 250:332–347

8. Jung J, Zheng M, Goldfarb M, Zaret KS (1999) Initiation of mammalian liver development from endoderm by fibroblast growth factors. Science 284:1998–2003

9. Zaret KS (2000) Liver specification and early morphogenesis. Mech Dev 92:83–88

10. Kamiya A, Kinoshita T, Ito Y, Matsui T, Morikawa Y, Senba E, Nakashima K, Taga T, Yoshida K, Kishimoto T, Miyajima A (1999) Fetal liver development requires a paracrine action of oncostatin M through the gp130 signal transducer. EMBO J 18:2127–2136

11. Davis RJ (2000) Signal transduction by the JNK group of MAP kinases. Cell 103:239–252

12. Chang L, Karin M (2001) Mammalian MAP kinase signaling cascades. Nature 410:37–40

13. Nishina H, Fischer KD, Radvanyi L, Shahinian A, Hakem R, Rubie EA, Bernstein A, Mak TW, Woodgett JR, Penninger JM (1997) Stress-signalling kinase Sek1 protects thymocytes from apoptosis mediated by CD95 and CD3. Nature 385:350–353

14. Nishina H, Bachmann M, Oliveira-dos-Santos AJ, Kozieradzki I, Fischer KD, Odermatt B, Wakeham A, Shahinian A, Takimoto H, Bernstein A, Mak TW, Woodgett JR, Ohashi PS, Penninger JM (1997) Impaired CD28-mediated interleukin 2 production and proliferation in stress kinase SAPK/ERK1 kinase (SEK1)/mitogen-activated protein kinase kinase4 (MKK4)-deficient T lymphocytes. J Exp Med 186:941–953

15. Nishina H, Vaz C, Billia P, Nghiem M, Sasaki T, Pompa JL, Furlonger K, Paige C, Hui CC, Fischer KD, Kishimoto H, Iwatsubo T, Katada T, Woodgett JR, Penninger JM (1999) Defective liver formation and liver cell apoptosis in mice lacking the stress signaling kinase SEK1/MKK4. Development 126:505–516

16. Yang D, Tournier C, Wysk M, Lu HT, Xu J, Davis RJ, Flavell RA (1997) Targeted disruption of the MKK4 gene causes embryonic death, inhibition of c-Jun NH2-terminal kinase activation, and defects in AP-1 transcriptional activity. Proc Natl Acad Sci USA 94:3004–3009

17. Ganiatsas S, Kwee L, Fujiwara Y, Perkins A, Ikeda T, Labow MA, Zon LI (1998) SEK1 deficiency reveals mitogen-activated protein kinase cascade crossregulation and leads to abnormal hepatogenesis. Proc Natl Acad Sci USA 95:6881–6886

18. Hilberg F, Aguzzi A, Howells N, Wagner EF (1993) c-Jun is essential for normal mouse development and hepatogenesis. Nature 365:179–181

19. Johnson RS, van Lingen B, Papaioannou VE, Spiegelman BM (1993) A null mutation at the *c-jun* locus causes embryonic lethality and retarded cell growth in culture. Genes Dev 7:1309–1317

20. Liu ZG, Hsu H, Goeddel DV, Karin M (1996) Dissection of TNF receptor 1 effector functions: JNK activation is not linked to apoptosis while NF-κB activation prevents cell death. Cell 87:565–576

21. Beg AA, Sha WC, Bronson RT, Ghosh S, Baltimore D (1995) Embryonic lethality and liver degeneration in mice lacking the RelA component of NF-κB. Nature 376:167–170

22. Li Q, Van Antwerp D, Mercurio F, Lee K-F, Verma IM (1999) Severe liver degeneration in mice lacking the IκB kinase 2 gene. Science 284:321–325

23. Li ZW, Chu W, Hu Y, Delhase M, Deerinck T, Ellisman M, Johnson R, Karin M (1999) The IKKβ subunit of IκB kinase (IKK) is essential for NF-κB activation and prevention of apoptosis. J Exp Med 189:1839–1845

24. Tanaka M, Fuentes ME, Yamaguchi K, Durnin MH, Dalrymple SA, Hardy KL, Goeddel DV (1999) Embryonic lethality, liver degeneration and impaired NF-κB activation in IKK-β-deficient mice. Immunity 10:421–429

25. Rudolph D, Yeh W-C, Wakeham A, Rudolph B, Nallainathan D, Potter J, Elia AJ, Mak TW (2000) Severe liver degeneration and lack of NF-κB activation in NEMO/IKKγ-deficient mice. Genes Dev 14:854–862

26. Bonnard M, Mirtsos C, Suzuki S, Graham K, Huang J, Ng M, Itie A, Wakeham A, Shahinian A, Henzel WJ, Elia AJ, Shillinglaw W, Mak TW, Cao Z, Yeh W-C (2000) Deficiency of T2K leads to apoptotic liver degeneration and impaired NF-κB-dependent gene transcription. EMBO J 19:4976–4985

27. Rosenfeld ME, Prichard L, Shiojiri N, Fausto N (2000) Prevention of hepatic apoptosis and embryonic lethality in RelA/TNFR-1 double knockout mice. Am J Pathol 156:997–1007

28. Okuda T, van Deursen J, Hiebert SW, Grosveld G, Downing JR (1996) AML1, the target of multiple chromosomal translocations in human leukemia, is essential for normal fetal liver hematopoiesis. Cell 84:321–330

29. Wang Q, Stacy T, Binder M, Marin-Padilla M, Sharpe AH, Speck NA (1996) Disruption of the *Cbfa2* gene causes necrosis and hemorrhaging in the central nervous system and blocks definitive hematopoiesis. Proc Natl Acad Sci USA 93:3444–3449

30. Eferl R, Sibilia M, Hilberg F, Fuchsbichler A, Kufferath I, Guertl B, Zenz R, Wagner EF, Zatloukal K (1999) Functions of c-Jun in liver and heart development. J Cell Biol 145:1049–1061

31. Gendron RL, Nestel FP, Lapp WS, Baines MG (1990) Lipopolysaccharide-induced fetal resorption in mice is associated with the intrauterine production of tumour necrosis factor-alpha. J Reprod Fertil 90:395–402

32. Haddad EK, Duclos AJ, Lapp WS, Baines MG (1997) Early embryo loss is associated with the prior expression of macrophage activation markers in the decidua. J Immunol 15:4886–4892

33. Lea RG, McIntyre S, Baird JD, Clark DA (1998) Tumor necrosis factor-alpha mRNA-positive cells in spontaneous resorption in rodents. Am J Reprod Immunol 39:50–57

34. Hamazaki T, Iiboshi Y, Oka M, Papst PJ, Meacham AM, Zon LI, Terada N (2001) Hepatic maturation in differentiating embryonic stem cells in vitro. FEBS Lett 497:15–19

35. Wada T, Nakagawa K, Watanabe T, Nishitai G, Seo J, Kishimoto H, Kitagawa D, Sasaki T, Penninger JM, Nishina H, Katada T (2001) Impaired synergistic-activation of stress-activated protein kinase SAPK/JNK in mouse embryonic stem cells lacking SEK1/MKK4. J Biol Chem 276:30892–30897

36. Sasaki T, Wada T, Kishimoto H, Irie-Sasaki J, Matsumoto G, Goto T, Yao Z, Wakeham A, Mak TW, Suzuki A, Katada T, Nishina H, Penninger JM (2001) The stress kinase MKK7 is a negative regulator of antigen receptor and growth factor receptor induced proliferation in hematopoietic cells. J Exp Med 194:757–768

37. Matsumoto K, Yoshitomi H, Rossant J, Zaret KS (2001) Liver organogenesis promoted by endothelial cells prior to vascular function. Science 294:559–563

38. Grisham JW, Thorgeirsson SS (1997) Liver stem cells. In: Potten CS (ed) Stem Cells. Academic, pp 233–282

39. Mittrucker HW, Pfeffer K, Schmits R, Mak TW (1996) T-lymphocyte development and function in gene-targeted mutant mice. Stem Cells 14:250–268

40. Schmidt C, Bladt F, Goedecke S, Brinkmann V, Zschiesche W, Sharpe M, Gherardi E, Birchmeire C (1995) Scatter factor/hepatocye growth factor is essential for liver development. Nature 373:699–702

41. Uehara Y, Minowa O, Mori C, Shiota K, Kuno J, Noda T, Kitamura N (1995) Placental defect and embryonic lethality in mice lacking hepatocyte growth factor/scatter factor. Nature 373:702–705
42. Kuan CY, Yang DD, Samanta Roy DR, Davis RJ, Rakic P, Flavell RA (1999) The Jnk1 and Jnk2 protein kinases are required for regional specific apoptosis during early brain development. Neuron 22:667–676

Promising Resources of Hepatic Progenitor Cells

Sei Kakinuma[1], Ryoko Chinzei[1], and Yujiro Tanaka[2]

Summary. Allogeneic liver transplantation remains the only effective treatment available to patients with liver failure. Because of a serious shortage of liver donors, however, an alternative therapeutic approach is urgently needed. It would be beneficial if we could obtain functional hepatocytes from nonhepatic sources to utilize for cell transplantation. Embryonic stem (ES) cells and umbilical cord blood (UCB) cells may have advantages as grafts for cell transplantation, because of their immaturity and plasticity. In contrast to their hematopoietic and mesenchymal potential, it remains unclear whether these cells function as endodermal epithelial cells. Here, with a view to utilizing ES cells and UCB cells for cell transplantation into injured liver, we investigated the hepatic potential of these types of cells both in vitro and in vivo. In the experiments with ES cells, mouse ES-derived embryoid bodies (EBs) cells were shown to contain functional hepatocytes, displaying a capacity to synthesize urea in vitro. After EB cells were transplanted relatively early in their differentiation in vitro, even before expressing hepatocyte phenotypes, they continued to differentiate into functional hepatocytes in vivo. In the experiments with UCB cells, human UCB cells proliferated and gave rise to hepatocyte-lineage cells in our original primary culture system. Also, human UCB-derived cells displayed the capacity to differentiate into functional hepatocytes in the liver after cell transplantation. In conclusion, this study demonstrates that ES cells and UCB cells could be promising resources of transplantable hepatic progenitor cells. Our findings may have relevance to the clinical application of ES-derived or UCB-derived cell transplantation as a novel therapeutic option for liver failure.

Key words. Embryonic stem cells, Umbilical cord blood, Hepatocyte, Albumin, Cell transplantation

Introduction

The survival of patients with fulminant hepatic failure is 15% to 25% [1]. Liver transplantation is currently the only established successful treatment for acute hepatic failure or endstage liver disease. However, the severe scarcity of donor organs has

[1]Department of Gastroenterology and Hepatology, [2]Department of General Medicine, Tokyo Medical and Dental University, 1-5-45 Yushima, Bunkyo-ku, Tokyo 113-8519, Japan

become a major limitation. Hepatocyte transplantation may partially solve this problem. Nevertheless, this treatment still requires the liver from a donor, and needs invasive surgical procedures [2]. Accordingly, it would be greatly beneficial if we could produce functional hepatocytes from nonhepatic sources, including embryonic stem (ES) cells, bone marrow (BM)-derived cells, or umbilical cord blood (UCB) cells.

ES cells are continuously growing stem-cell lines of embryonic origin first isolated from the inner cell mass of developing blastocysts [3–5]. When ES cells are allowed to differentiate under appropriate conditions in vitro, the cells form structures called embryoid bodies (EBs) that are similar to embryos of the egg cylinder stage. EBs are composed of an outer endodermal layer, which is like the primitive endoderm of the embryo, and an inner ectodermal layer homologous to the primitive ectoderm. At a later stage, EBs consist of multiple differentiated cell types, including hematopoietic, cardiac muscle, neuronal, insulin-producing, and yolk-sac cells. Recently, mouse ES cells have been suggested to have the potential to differentiate into hepatocytes in vitro, on the basis of reverse transcription-polymerase chain reaction (RT-PCR) analysis of hepatic genes [6]. Additional experiments would be required to examine liver-specific functions, such as the production of albumin (ALB) and the synthesis of urea.

UCB contains circulating stem/progenitor cells, and the cellular contents of UCB are known to be quite distinct from those of BM and adult peripheral blood. The frequency of hematopoietic stem/progenitor cells in UCB equals or exceeds that in BM and greatly surpasses that in adult peripheral blood [7]. Compared with adult cells, UCB hematopoietic stem cells produce larger hematopoietic colonies in vitro, have different growth-factor requirements, are able to expand in longterm culture in vitro, and have longer telomeres [8]. UCB transplantation for various hematopoietic diseases has resulted in successful hematopoietic reconstitution and a lower incidence of graft-versus-host disease than expected with conventional therapies [9]. Recently, it has been reported that UCB contains mesenchymal progenitor cells capable of differentiating into marrow stroma, bone, cartilage, muscle, and connective tissues [10]. Furthermore, UCB gives rise to no ethical problems for basic studies and clinical applications. UCB cells can be collected without any harm to the newborn infant, and UCB hematopoietic stem-cell grafts can be cryopreserved and transplanted to a host after thawing without losing their repopulating ability. For these reasons, UCB could be a prominent source of cells for transplantation in various diseases. It remains obscure, however, whether UCB contains stem/progenitor cells that lead to endodermal cells, including hepatocytes.

Most recently, we have demonstrated the differentiation of mouse ES cells and human UCB cells into functional hepatocytes in both in vitro and in vivo models [11,12]. At first, in the study of ES cells, we found that cultured EBs derived from an ES cell line contained functional hepatocytes displaying the capacity for urea synthesis in vitro, and that EBs differentiated into mature hepatocytes in vivo. Then, in the study of UCB cells, we found that UCB cells proliferated and gave rise to hepatocyte-lineage cells in vitro, and that human UCB cells displayed the characteristics of functionally differentiated hepatocytes in vivo. Therefore, ES cells and UCB cells could be promising resources of transplantable hepatic cells for the treatment of liver injury.

Materials and Methods

Culture of ES Cells and EBs

Mouse ES cells (BL6 cell line, derived from male C57/BL6 mouse-embryo) were kindly provided by Dr. Naohiro Terada, University of Florida. Undifferentiated ES cells were maintained in KNOCKOUT DMEM containing 20% KNOCKOUT serum replacement (GIBCO-BRL, Grand Island, NY, USA), 300 μM monothioglycerol, 2 mM L-glutamine, 100 U/ml penicillin, 100 μg/ml streptomycin, and 25 mM hydroxyethylpiperazine ethanesulfonic acid (HEPES). The medium was supplemented with 1000 U/ml recombinant mouse leukemia inhibitory factor (LIF). To induce differentiation, ES cells were suspended in IMDM containing 15% fetal calf serum (FCS), 300 μM monothioglycerol, 2 mM L-glutamine, 100 U/ml penicillin, and 100 μg/ml streptomycin without LIF.

Culture of UCB Cells

UCB samples from full-term deliveries were collected after informed consent in writing had been obtained. The study protocol was approved by the ethics committees of the Medical Research Institute, Tokyo Medical and Dental University, and Kanto Medical Center NTT EC. Equal volumes of UCB and 6% hydroxyethylstarch were mixed in sterile centrifuge tubes, and left to stand for 90 min. The red cells were allowed to settle by gravity. Nucleated cells were obtained from the supernatant. After one washing with sterilized phosphate-buffered saline (PBS), isolated UCB cells were primarily cultured in DMEM supplemented with 15% FCS, 2 mM L-glutamine, 25 mM HEPES, 100 U/ml penicillin, 100 μg/ml streptomycin, 0.25 μg/ml amphotericin B, 300 μM monothioglycerol, and a combination of several growth/differentiation factors, including recombinant human fibroblast growth factor (FGF), recombinant human LIF, recombinant human stem cell factor (SCF), recombinant human hepatocyte growth factor (HGF), recombinant human oncostatin M (OSM), and dexamethasone.

Analysis of Hepatocyte-Lineage Markers in Cultured Cells

Hepatocyte-lineage markers in cultured cells were detected by use of RT-PCR and Western blot analysis. The cultured cells were collected after treatment with 0.25% trypsin-ethylenediamine tetraacetic acid (EDTA) for further analysis. Total RNA was extracted from the cultured cells, and first-strand cDNA was synthesized using Superscript II RNase H reverse transcriptase (GIBCO-BRL) according to the manufacturer's instructions. The resulting cDNA was amplified by PCR. PCR primers for mouse glyceraldehyde 3-phosphate dehydrogenase (GAPDH), mouse ALB, mouse Oct-3/4, mouse tyrosine aminotransferase (TAT), human GAPDH, human ALB, human alpha-fetoprotein (AFP), human cytokeratin (CK)-18, human alpha-1-antitrypsin (AAT), and human glutamine synthetase (GS) were synthesized based on the reported sequences. For Western blot analysis, a goat anti-rat ALB antibody (ICN Biomedicals, Aurora, OH, USA) and an anti-human ALB (clone 4761; Institute of Immunology, Tokyo, Japan) monoclonal antibody (mAb) were used as primary antibodies.

Immunofluorescent Staining Analysis of the Cultured Cells

Cultured cells were fixed with 80% acetone for 20 min at −20°C. Samples were washed three times with PBS, then incubated for 1 h with diluted primary antibodies at room temperature. Goat anti-rat ALB antibody (ICN Biomedicals), rabbit anti-human ALB antibody (DAKO, Kyoto, Japan), anti-human CK-18 mAb (clone DC10; DAKO), and anti-human CK-19 mAb (clone IF15; Oncogene Research Products, Cambridge, MA, USA) were used. Samples were washed three times with PBS, then incubated for 30 min at room temperature with appropriate secondary antibodies.

Cell Transplantation

C57/BL6 female mice and C.B-17/Icr severe combined immunodeficiency (SCID) mice were purchased. They were given one subcutaneous injection of 0.4 mg/body 2-acetylaminofluorene (2-AAF), then, 7 days after the injection, they were subjected to one-third partial hepatectomy and the infusion of a total of 5×10^5 isolated ES or EB cells (to C57/BL6 female mice), or a total of 1×10^7 isolated UCB cells (C.B-17/Icr SCID mice) in 0.1 ml of PBS into the liver via the portal vein, under anesthesia. Control mice were subjected only to 2-AAF injection and partial hepatectomy. These mice were killed 4 to 55 weeks after cell transplantation. The animals were managed according to Tokyo Medical and Dental University guidelines.

Fluorescence in situ Hybridization (FISH) and Immunohistochemical Staining of the Liver Tissues of Recipient Mice

Liver tissues of the recipient mice were subjected to FISH and immunostaining as described previously [11,12]. Goat anti-rat ALB antibody (ICN Biomedicals), rabbit anti-human ALB (DAKO), and anti-human hepatocyte mAb (clone OCH1E5; DAKO) were used as the primary antibody. Biotinylated probe for mouse Y-chromosome (Applied Genetics Laboratories, Melbourne, FL, USA) and human X chromosome labeled with fluorescein isothiocyanate (FITC) (Vysis, Downers Grove, IL, USA) were used in the FISH procedure, and were treated according to the manufacturer's instructions.

Results

Expression of ALB in the Cultured EBs

At first, to assess the differentiation of mouse ES cells into hepatic lineages, we examined the mRNA and protein expressions of liver-specific markers, including ALB. ES cells were incubated by the hanging-drop culture method and formed EBs in hanging drops (Fig. 1). After 2 days of culture in the differentiation medium, EBs were plated on tissue culture plates, and allowed to attach and spread in further culture. First, the steady-state level of ALB, AFP, and TAT mRNAs was determined, by RT-PCR, in mouse ES cells and in differentiating EBs every 3 days without exogenous growth factors. AFP represents endodermal differentiation as well as being an early fetal hepatic marker, and its expression decreases as the liver develops. AFP was expressed from

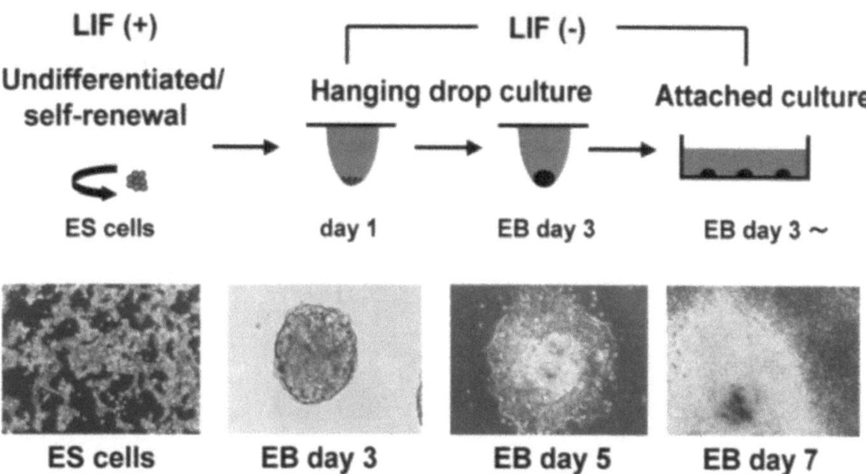

Fig. 1. Formation of embryoid bodies (*EBs*) from embryonic stem (*ES*) cell line. ES cells were incubated by the hanging-drop culture method and formed EBs in hanging drops. After 2 days of culture in the differentiation medium, EBs were plated on tissue culture plates, and allowed to attach and spread in further culture. *LIF*, leukemia inhibitory factor

day 9 and was maintained throughout the culture up to day 21. ALB mRNA appeared in EBs on day 12, and increased with the culture period of EBs, whereas no mRNA expression of ALB and AFP was seen in ES cells. TAT was also expressed on day 12 or later. These results were similar to those in the previous report [6]. Although several growth/differentiation factors, including FGF, HGF, and OSM were added to the culture media of EBs, there was no significant effect on the mRNA expression of ALB, AFP, and TAT. Next, we examined ALB protein, a liver-specific protein, by Western blot analysis. ALB protein first appeared on day 15 following ALB mRNA expression on day 12, and the level reached maximum on day 18. These data suggest that ES cells have the potential to differentiate into hepatocyte lineage in vitro. Similarly to the results of the RT-PCR analysis of ALB mRNA, Western blot analysis of ALB in EBs did not show any significant change in the presence of exogenous growth factors.

Then, EBs on day 21, which expressed ALB protein, were immunostained. ALB-producing cells were seen in the stratiform cells rather than in monolayer cells. Only some cells in cultured EBs showed an ALB positive area, which was in the cytoplasm. These results showed that hepatocyte-like, ALB-producing cells appeared when EBs derived from the ES cell line were adherently cultured for differentiation.

Urea Synthesis by the Cultured EBs

We investigated the urea synthetic ability of EBs from the point of view of hepatocyte-specific function. Substantial synthesis of urea in EBs was first observed on day 12, and the level reached maximum on day 18, while, for up to 9 days, ES cells and cultured EBs produced no comparable synthesis of urea. The time course of urea synthesis seemed to be roughly parallel to that of ALB protein expression.

Table 1. Formation of teratomas by transplantation with ES cells and EBs

	Incidence of teratomas[a]	
Cell type	Liver	Spleen
Dissociated		
ES cell	86% (6/7)	86% (6/7)
ES day 2	75% (3/4)	75% (3/4)
ES day 4	40% (2/5)	60% (3/5)
ES day 6	20% (2/10)	50% (5/10)
ES day 9	0% (0/10)	20% (2/10)
Nondissociated		
ES day 15	89%(8/9)	ND

ES cell, embryonic stem cell; EB, embryoid body; ND, not determined

[a]Incidence of teratoma formation in recipient mice transplanted with ES cells and dissociated cells from EBs

Incidence of Teratoma in EB-Transplanted Liver

We investigated whether or not the incidence of teratoma in recipient mice was dependent on the culture period of the transplanted EBs. In recipient mice transplanted with ES cells, typical teratomas were seen in the spleen and the liver, but the incidence decreased with the culture period. Finally, no teratoma was found in the liver of mice transplanted with dissociated cells from day-9 EBs (Table 1).

For comparison, we transplanted nondissociated EBs in 15-day culture, which expressed ALB protein and synthesized urea. We were able to prepare dissociated cells from day-9 EBs by trypsin treatment, but it was difficult to trypsinize day-12 or later EBs into dissociated cells. Interestingly, we observed a very high incidence of teratoma formation with the nondissociated EBs in 15-day culture. This suggests the importance of the microenvironment of engrafted cells, in addition to their stage of differentiation.

Transplanted Cells in the Recipient Liver

We investigated whether the dissociated cells from EBs could differentiate into hepatocytes when they were transplanted via the portal vein to the liver. We employed day-9 EBs as a source of dissociated cells for transplantation into liver, because no teratoma appeared in the liver of recipient mice 4 weeks after the transplantation. The liver tissues were examined to identify which cells were derived from male ES cells containing the Y chromosome and also produced ALB. In the livers of female mice who were transplanted with dissociated cells from day-9 EBs, EB-derived cells were identified, based on the presence of the Y chromosome within their nuclei, and ALB expression was also seen in their cytoplasm (Fig. 2). According to our observation, almost all Y-chromosome-positive cells were also ALB-positive. These results indicated that dissociated cells from day-9 EBs are capable of differentiating into ALB-producing cells in the recipient liver in mice.

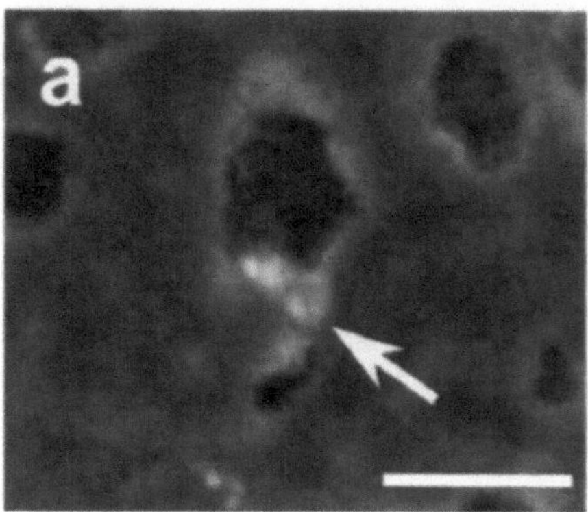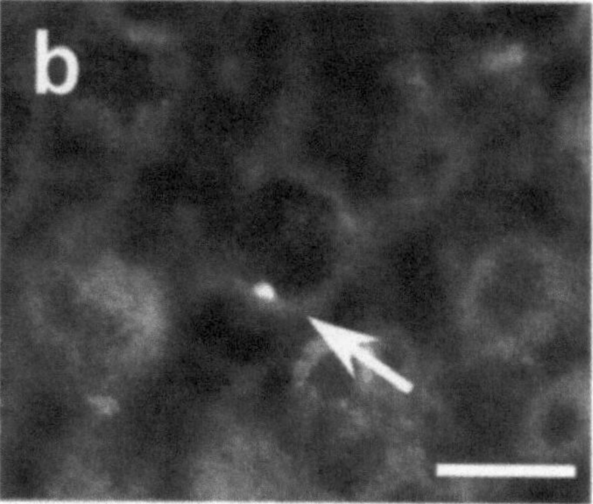

Fig. 2a,b. Immunohistochemical staining for albumin (ALB) and fluorescence in situ hybridization (FISH) for Y chromosome in the recipient mouse liver. Confocal microscopic images of liver obtained from female mice 4 weeks after the transplantation. Two representative pictures are shown. ES-derived cells were identified among recipient hepatocytes, based on the presence of the Y chromosome within their nuclei, and ALB expression was seen in their cytoplasm. Both Y-chromosome- and ALB-positive cells are hepatocytes derived from EB cells (*arrows*). *Scale bars*, 10 μm, ×1000

Expression of ALB in the Cultured UCB Cells

Next, in order to investigate the hepatic competence of UCB cells in vitro, we established a novel primary culture system. Nucleated cells isolated from UCB were cultured in the basic medium supplemented with various combinations of growth/differentiation factors (FGF-1, FGF-2, LIF, SCF, HGF, and OSM), each of which contributes in a different manner to the proliferation and differentiation of hepatic progenitor cells in the livers of rodents and humans [13–17]. We compared the effects of 34 different combinations or sequential additions of FGF-1, FGF-2, LIF, SCF, HGF, and OSM. Human ALB mRNA was detected at the highest level in the cultured cells with the combination of FGF-1, FGF-2, LIF, SCF, and HGF, and was detectable in 75% of samples from different donors. On the basis of these examinations, we determined that this combination was the most efficient in leading UCB cells to express ALB mRNA.

We examined the time-dependency of the ALB mRNA expression and the production of ALB in the UCB cells. RT-PCR analysis indicated the expression of ALB mRNA in the 7-day culture of UCB cells, and increased expression was observed at 14 and 21 days, whereas no transcript of ALB was detected on day 0. Quantitative RT-PCR analysis showed that the ALB mRNA level of the 21-day cultured cells was about 40-fold higher than that of the 7-day cultured cells. From the morphological viewpoint, small round cells appeared at 7 days, and both round and spindle-shaped cells were observed at 14 and 21 days. Immunofluorescent staining analysis demonstrated that the round cells, but not the spindle-shaped cells, expressed ALB (Fig. 3), and the number of ALB-producing round cells increased with the culture period. ALB-positive cells accounted for about 50% of the attached cells at 21 days in the primary culture. These results demonstrate that UCB cells cultured with the combination of

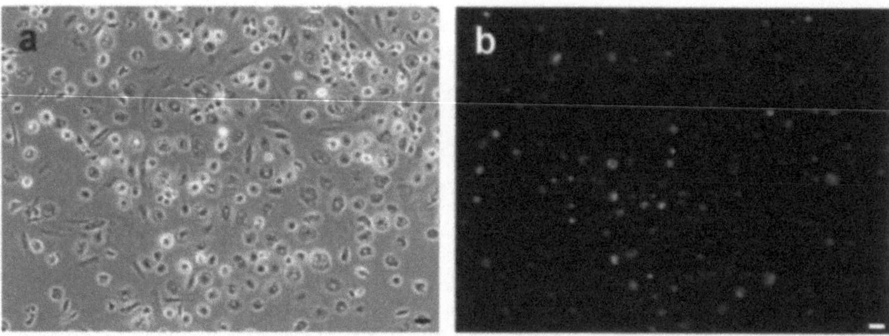

Fig. 3a,b. ALB expression and morphology of 21-day cultured umbilical cord blood (UCB) cells. **a** Phase-contrast view and **b** immunofluorescent staining of ALB with fluorescein isothiocyanate(FITC)-labeled anti-rabbit IgG antibody in the cultured UCB cells. The round cells, but not the spindle-shaped cells, expressed ALB. ALB-positive cells (*white cells in* **b**) accounted for about 50% of the attached cells. *Scale bars*, 10 μm, ×100

FGF-1, FGF-2, LIF, SCF, and HGF are capable of giving rise to ALB-producing cells efficiently in vitro.

Expression Profiles of Hepatocyte-Lineage Markers

To confirm that the cultured cells derived from UCB give rise to the hepatocyte lineage, we examined additional differentiation markers for hepatocyte lineages. RT-PCR analysis revealed that transcripts of AFP, CK-18, and GS were expressed in the 21-day cultured cells. Next, immunofluorescent analysis showed that the cultured cells expressed CK-19. CK-19 is a cell marker for bile duct epithelial cells and hepatic progenitor cells, such as "oval cells" [18]. Dual-immunostaining analysis indicated that ALB was co-expressed with CK-19 in some cultured round cells. Co-expression of ALB and CK-19 demonstrated that these double-positive cells derived from UCB had the same character as bipotential hepatic progenitor cells. Taken together, the expression profiles of ALB, AFP, CK-18, GS, and CK-19 show that various stages of the hepatocyte lineage, including both hepatic progenitor cells and mature hepatocytes, are present in our cultured UCB cells. It is reasonable to consider that UCB cells differentiated into mature hepatocytes via hepatic stem cells in our primary culture system.

UCB-Derived Hepatocytes in the Livers of the Recipient Mice

To investigate whether UCB is a potential source of transplantable cells for the treatment of liver injury, cell transplantation was performed in liver-injured SCID mice. We traced human UCB-derived parenchymal cells by immunostaining analysis against human hepatocyte-specific antigen. In human liver samples, almost all hepatocytes and bile duct cells, but not other nonparenchymal cells, were stained with the antibody, and no cells were stained in the control mouse liver. Figure 4 shows UCB-derived parenchymal cells in the liver of mice killed at 4 weeks. UCB-derived cells

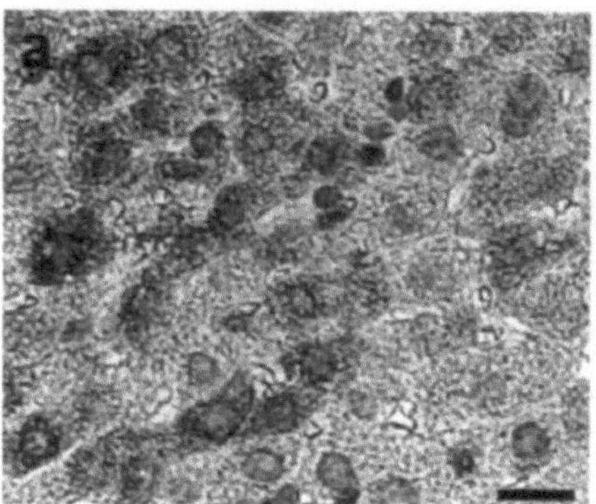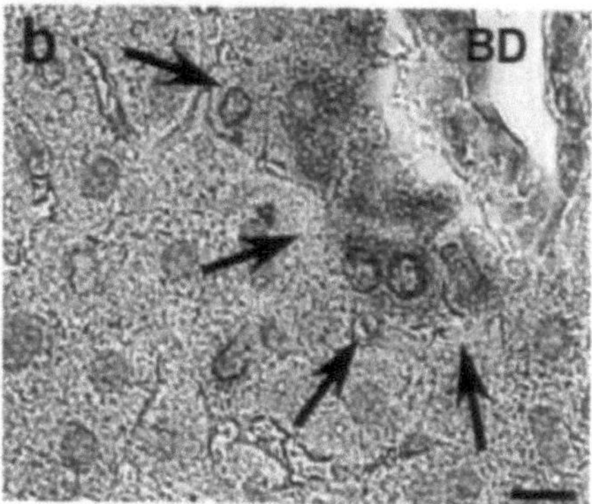

Fig. 4a,b. Human UCB-derived hepatocytes in the liver of recipient mice. Immunoperoxidase staining of liver obtained from recipient mice 4 weeks after the transplantation. Two representative pictures are shown. Human hepatocytes were detected by the use of anti-human hepatocyte monoclonal antibody. **a** UCB-derived cells (*dark cells*) were widely distributed in hepatic lobules. **b** A cluster of human UCB-derived parenchymal cells (*arrows*) was observed in the periportal area. *BD*, bile duct. *Scale bars*, 10 μm, ×400

were widely distributed in hepatic lobules (Fig. 4a). Clusters of more than ten parenchymal donor cells were observed in the livers of mice at 4 weeks (Fig. 4b). Moreover, UCB-derived parenchymal cells were detected in the livers of mice sacrificed 55 weeks after transplantation. These data indicated that human hepatocytes derived from UCB have the ability to form longterm engraftment even in xenogeneic conditions.

In order to evaluate the function of these repopulating cells, we analyzed the production of ALB in the UCB-derived parenchymal cells. Double-immunofluorescent staining with anti-human hepatocyte and anti-human ALB antibodies demonstrated that UCB-derived parenchymal cells produced human ALB in the recipient-mouse liver. These double-positive cells were observed even 55 weeks after inoculation. Furthermore, we detected human ALB in the sera of the recipient mice by use of Western blot analysis. These observations prove that inoculated UCB cells developed into functional hepatocytes, and that UCB-derived hepatocytes may play a role in the support for liver injury.

Discussion

In this study, we provided, for the first time, direct evidence that mouse ES cells and human UCB cells differentiate into functional hepatocytes not only in vitro but also in vivo [11,12]. When ES cells are transplanted into a mouse, teratoma develops, then becomes greater, and finally kills the recipient mouse [4]. Therefore, we examined the relationship between the culture period of EBs employed for transplantation and the incidence of teratoma in the livers of the mice. Teratomas were frequently seen in the livers of mice which had been transplanted with ES cells via the portal vein, but the incidence of teratoma decreased with the culture period of EBs, and no teratoma was found in the livers of mice transplanted with dissociated cells from day-9 EBs. In addition, when we utilized nondissociated day-15 EBs for transplantation, teratomas were frequently seen in the recipient liver, at an incidence similar to that seen with ES cells (Table 1). These results suggested that the probability of teratoma formation in the recipient liver was affected by both the grade of differentiation of ES-derived cells in vitro and the microenvironment of the implanted cells. On the other hand, even at 55 weeks after the transplantation of UCB cells, there was no formation of tumors in the liver, such as teratomas. This result implied that we could utilize UCB for cell transplantation without risk of tumor.

Recently, BM cells have been reported to have the potential for differentiation into multilineage cells, including hepatocytes, in both in vitro and in vivo models [19–21]. BM-derived multipotent adult progenitor cells (MAPCs) [21] are possible resources for cell transplantation if they can proliferate quickly in vitro or in the target organ. The advantage of utilizing MAPCs is that the transplants would be obtained from autologous cells. However, the establishment of MAPCs from BM, with the use of numerous growth/differentiation factors, would be expensive. Moreover, the utilization of human BM as an allogeneic graft source is restricted by the shortage of healthy donors. We are not able to use ES cells and UCB cells without restriction as well as the use of BM cells. The clinical application of human ES cells obtained from human fertilized eggs involves serious ethical problems in many countries. A method for avoiding ES-cell-derived teratoma formation should be established. In the case of UCB cells, a more efficient method for expanding UCB-derived hepatocytes on a large scale would be needed. Furthermore, in regard to each of these cell types, ES, UCB, and BM, it is still unclear whether hepatocytes derived from these extrahepatic resources could actually improve liver function in disease model mice in which allogeneic hepatocyte transplantation is known to be effective.

Allogeneic liver transplantation, however, has an advantage over other organ transplantation procedures, because graft rejection is rather moderate. Kidney transplantation or BM transplantation requires HLA matching, while liver transplantation requires only ABO blood type compatibility. Therefore, this loose restriction against graft rejection may lead us to a cell-transplantation procedure for the treatment of liver injury, if we can prepare enough liver cells to improve liver function. When we can successfully utilize ES-derived or UCB-derived hepatocytes as a source of cell transplantation for decompensated liver diseases, we should be able to overcome the problems of the short supply of organs in liver transplantation.

References

1. Bernuau J, Rueff B, Benhamou JP (1986) Fulminant and subfulminant hepatic failure: definition and causes. Semin Liver Dis 6:97–106
2. Fox IJ, Chowdhury JR, Kaufman SS, Goertzen TC, Chowdhury NR, Warkentin PI, Dorko K, Sauter BV, Strom SC (1998) Treatment of the Crigler–Najjar syndrome type I with hepatocyte transplantation. N Engl J Med 338:1422–1427
3. Evans MJ, Kaufman MH (1981) Establishment in culture of pluripotent cells from mouse embryos. Nature 292:154–156
4. Martin GR (1981) Isolation of a pluripotent cell line from early mouse embryos cultured in medium conditioned by teratocarcinoma stem cells. Proc Natl Acad Sci USA 78:7634–7638

5. Thomson JA, Itskovitz-Eldor J, Shapiro SS, Waknitz MA, Swiergiel JJ, Marshall VS, Jones JM (1998) Embryonic stem cell lines derived from human blastocysts. Science 282:1145–1147

6. Hamazaki T, Iiboshi Y, Oka M, Papst PJ, Meacham AM, Zon LI, Terada N (2001) Hepatic maturation in differentiating embryonic stem cells in vitro. FEBS Lett 497:15–19

7. Mayani H, Lansdorp PM (1998) Biology of human umbilical cord blood-derived hematopoietic stem/progenitor cells. Stem Cells 16:153–165

8. Gluckman E (2000) Current status of umbilical cord blood hematopoietic stem cell transplantation. Exp Hematol 28:1197–1205

9. Kurtzberg J, Laughlin M, Graham ML, Smith C, Olson JF, Halperin EC, Ciocci G, Carrier C, Stevens CE, Rubinstein P (1996) Placental blood as a source of hematopoietic stem cells for transplantation into unrelated recipients. N Engl J Med 335:157–166

10. Erices A, Conget P, Minguell JJ (2000) Mesenchymal progenitor cells in human umbilical cord blood. Br J Hematol 109:235–242

11. Chinzei R, Tanaka Y, Shimizu-Saito K, Hara Y, Kakinuma S, Watanabe M, Teramoto K, Arii S, Takase K, Sato C, Terada N, Teraoka H (2002) Embryoid-body cells derived from a mouse embryonic stem cell line show differentiation into functional hepatocytes. Hepatology 36:22–29

12. Kakinuma S, Tanaka Y, Chinzei R, Watanabe M, Shimizu-Saito K, Hara Y, Teramoto K, Arii S, Sato C, Takase K, Yasumizu T, Teraoka H (2003). Human umbilical cord blood as a source of transplantable hepatic progenitor cells. Stem Cells 21:217–227

13. Jung J, Zheng M, Goldfarb M, Zaret KS (1999) Initiation of mammalian liver development from endoderm by fibroblast growth factor. Science 284:1998–2003

14. Baumann H, Zeigler SF, Mosley B, Morella KK, Pajovic S, Gearing DP (1993) Reconstitution of the response to leukemia inhibitory factor, oncostatin M and ciliary neurotrophic factor in hepatoma cells. J Biol Chem 268:8414–8417

15. Baumann U, Crosby HA, Ramani P, Kelly DA, Strain AJ (1999) Expression of the stem cell factor receptor c-kit in normal and diseased pediatric liver: identification of a human hepatic progenitor cell. Hepatology 30:112–117

16. Schmidt C, Bladt F, Goedecke S, Brinkmann V, Zschiesche S, Sharpe M, Gherardi E, Birchmeier C (1995) Scatter factor/hepatocyte growth factor is essential for liver development. Nature 373:699–702

17. Kinoshita T, Sekiguchi T, Xu M, Kamiya A, Tsuji K, Nakahata T, Miyajima A (1999) Hepatic differentiation induced by oncostatin M attenuates fetal liver hematopoiesis. Proc Natl Acad Sci USA 96:7265–7270

18. Theise ND, Saxena R, Portmann BC, Thung SN, Yee H, Chiriboga L, Kumar A, Crawford JM (1999) The canals of Herring and hepatic stem cells in humans. Hepatology 30:1425–1433

19. Petersen BE, Bowen WC, Patrene KD, Mars WM, Sullivan AK, Murase N, Boggs SS, Greenberger JS, Goff JP (1999) Bone marrow as a potential source of hepatic oval cells. Science 284:1168–1170

20. Lagasse E, Connors H, Al-Dhalimy M, Reitzma M, Dohse M, Osborne L, Wang X, Finegold M, Weissman IL, Grompe M (2000) Purified hematopoietic stem cells can differentiate into hepatocytes in vivo. Nat Med 6:1229–1234

21. Jiang Y, Jahagirdar BN, Reinhardt RL, Schwarz RE, Keene CD, Ortiz-Gonzalez XR, Reyes M, Lenvik T, Lund T, Blackstad M, Du J, Aldrich S, Lisberg A, Low WC, Largaespada DA, Verfaillie CM (2002) Pluripotency of mesenchymal stem cells derived from adult cells. Nature 418:41–49

Oncostatin M Promotes Differentiation of Fetal Hepatocytes in vitro and Regulates Liver Regeneration in vivo

Koji Nakamura[1] and Atsushi Miyajima[1,2,3]

Summary. The development as well as regeneration of liver involves sequential biological events, such as cell proliferation, differentiation, and morphogenesis, in response to various extracellular stimuli. However, the molecular processes of liver development and regeneration remain largely unknown. We previously established a primary culture system using immature hepatocytes derived from mouse fetal liver at embryonic day 14. This culture system made it possible to investigate several extracellular signals that influence hepatic differentiation. Retrovirus-mediated gene transfer into the primary culture made it possible to analyze intracellular signal pathways required for hepatic differentiation. We found that oncostatin M (OSM), an interleukin (IL)-6 family cytokine, specifically induced hepatic differentiation. Fetal hepatocytes treated with OSM acquired various metabolic functions and exhibited changed morphology, similar to that of adult hepatocytes, i.e., they showed glycogen synthesis, ammonia clearance, albumin secretion, and detoxification. Moreover, sequential treatment of the cells with extracellular matrix (ECM) followed by OSM induced terminal differentiation of hepatocytes in vitro, as evidenced by the expression of tryptophan oxygenase (TO). Retrovirus-mediated gene transfer and analysis of fetal hepatocytes from Ras knockout mice revealed that the signal transducer and activator of transcription protein 3 (STAT3) and Ras pathways play a distinct role in hepatic differentiation. In addition, we recently generated OSM receptor (OSMR) knockout mice (OSMR$^{-/-}$) and found that OSM regulated hepatocyte proliferation as well as the remodeling of the ECM during liver regeneration. Thus, the present results indicate that OSM plays an important role in liver development in the fetus and in liver regeneration in adults.

Key words. Oncostatin M, STAT3, Knockout mouse, Liver development, Liver regeneration

[1]Stem Cell Regulation Project, Kanagawa Academy of Science and Technology (KAST), 907 Nogawa, Miyamae-ku, Kawasaki, Kanagawa 216-0001, Japan
[2]Institute of Molecular and Cellular Biosciences, The University of Tokyo, 1-1-1 Yayoi, Bunkyo-ku, Tokyo 113-0032, Japan
[3]CREST, Japan Science and Technology Corporation, 4-1-8 Honcho, Kawaguchi, Saitama 332-0012, Japan

Introduction

Oncostatin M (OSM) is a member of the interleukin (IL)-6 family of cytokines that includes IL-6, IL-11, leukemia inhibitory factor (LIF), ciliary neurotrophic factor, cardiotropin-1, and the novel neurotrophin-1/B-cell stimulating factor-3 [1]. These cytokines share the gp130 receptor subunit as a common signal transducer [1]. Mouse OSM receptor (OSMR) is composed of the OSM-specific β subunit and gp130 [2]. Ligand binding to the receptor complex activates the Janus family of tyrosine kinases (Jak1, Jak2, and Tyk2) and the activated Jaks, in turn, activate downstream pathways such as SH2 domain-containing phosphatase (SHP)-2 tyrosine phosphatase and signal transducer and activator of transcription protein 3 (STAT3). We previously reported various OSM-specific biological activities during mouse development, e.g., stimulation of the production of definitive hematopoietic progenitors in the aorta-gonad-mesonephros (AGM) region of embryonic day 11 (E11) mouse embryo [3] and stimulation of the proliferation of Sertoli cells in neonatal testes [4]. Interestingly, these biological effects are specific to OSM among the IL-6 family of cytokines.

Liver development proceeds through several stages. In mice, hepatic progenitors/hepatoblasts emerge from the foregut endoderm after stimulation with fibroblast growth factors (FGF 1, 2, and 8) derived from the adjacent cardiac mesoderm and form the liver bud at E8-9 [5]. Then, committed hepatoblasts proliferate vigorously and increase their mass during development. Fetal liver is known to be the major hematopoietic organ, but not a metabolic organ, in the mid- to late-fetus [1,6]. With embryonic development, the liver gradually loses its hematopoietic activity. Instead, during the late-fetal and neonatal stages, the liver initiates the expression of various metabolic enzymes, such as glucose-6-phosphatase (G6Pase) and tyrosine aminotransferase (TAT) and starts forming the architecture of the liver lobules [7,8]. Finally, terminal differentiation occurs after birth, and the fully matured liver expresses adult liver-specific enzymes such as tryptophan oxygenase (TO) [9]. These multistep maturation processes of the liver are regulated by various soluble factors, such as cytokines and hormones, extracellular matrices (ECMs), and cell-cell contacts. To investigate factors that promote fetal hepatocyte differentiation, we previously established a primary culture system using mouse embryonic day-14 (E14) fetal hepatocytes [10]. By using this culture system, we found that OSM specifically induced the differentiation of fetal hepatocytes. Consistent with results in vitro, gp130-deficient liver exhibited limited accumulation of glycogen and decreased expression of TAT, indicating an important role for gp130-mediated signaling during liver development. Retrovirus-mediated gene transfer of various mutant receptors and signaling molecules in this primary culture system demonstrated that STAT3 is essential for functional liver maturation and that K-Ras is required for the formation of the E-cadherin-based adherens junction in hepatocytes [11,12].

It is well known that the liver has a remarkable ability to regenerate in response to injury caused by partial hepatectomy, toxic exposure, or viral infection [13,14]. Liver parenchymal cells, hepatocytes, are normally in the quiescent G_0, phase but reenter the cell cycle following injury to quickly restore the mass, architecture, and function of the liver. A number of cytokines, such as hepatocyte growth factor (HGF), epidermal growth factor (EGF), transforming growth factor (TGF)-α, tumor necrosis factor (TNF)-α, and IL-6 have been implicated in regulating this complex phenomenon

[13,14]. An important role for IL-6 signaling, including the activation of STAT3 in the initial step of liver regeneration, has been shown in IL-6 knockout (IL-6$^{-/-}$) mice [15,16]. IL-6$^{-/-}$ livers exhibit impaired proliferative responses in hepatocytes during liver regeneration induced by partial hepatectomy and carbon tetrachloride (CCl$_4$)-mediated injury.

As we found that OSM stimulated the differentiation of fetal hepatocytes in vitro and that gp130$^{-/-}$ liver exhibited defects, we generated OSMR$^{-/-}$ mice by homologous recombination and investigated the role of OSM in vivo. In contrast to gp130$^{-/-}$ mice, OSMR$^{-/-}$ mice develop normally, suggesting that the functions of OSM in liver development are compensated by other IL-6 family cytokines in vivo. However, we have found that OSMR$^{-/-}$ mice exhibit impaired liver regeneration, i.e., delayed hepatocyte proliferation, persistent liver necrosis, and reduced expression of tissue inhibitor of metalloproteinase-1 (TIMP-1).

Here, we describe the functions of OSM in liver development and regeneration.

Role of OSM in Liver Development

OSM Promotes Fetal Hepatocyte Differentiation

Because mid-fetal liver is a major hematopoietic but not metabolic organ, fetal hepatocytes do not express differentiation marker genes such as *G6Pase* and *TAT*. Immature fetal hepatocytes proliferate vigorously and acquire various metabolic functions, such as the production of serum proteins, glycogen accumulation, ammonia clearance, and so on, with development. In order to find factors that promote fetal liver development and to investigate the molecular basis of fetal hepatic development, we previously established a primary culture system using fetal hepatocytes derived from E14 mouse embryo [9,10]. As fetal liver is a hematopoietic organ, more than 70% of fetal hepatic cells at this stage are hematopoietic cells. Fetal liver cells were dissociated with liver digestion medium (GIBCO-BRL, Gaithersburg, MD, USA) and plated on 0.1% gelatin-coated cell-culture dishes. Floating hematopoietic cells were washed out extensively and the remaining adhesive cells exhibited a morphology similar to that of epithelial cells, and they expressed alpha-fetoprotein, albumin, and hepatic nuclear factors (hepatocyte nuclear factor [HNF]-1, HNF-4), but not G6Pase or TAT, indicating that these cells were immature hepatocytes. This primary culture made it possible to search for a cytokine that stimulates fetal hepatocyte differentiation in vitro. Among the various cytokines examined, including IL-6, IL-11, LIF, OSM, and TGF-β, OSM specifically induced the gene expression of differentiation markers such as *G6Pase* and *TAT* in a dose- and time-dependent manner (Fig. 1). In addition to the expression of differentiation marker genes, OSM induced glycogenic activity and ammonia clearance [10,17]. Besides inducing the functional maturation, OSM induced morphological maturation as well. In the presence of OSM, a mature hepatocyte-like morphology was observed, e.g., tight cell-cell contact, highly condensed and granulated cytosol, and clear round nuclei (Fig. 1a). Ultrastructural analysis, using an electron microscope, revealed that fetal hepatocytes treated with OSM developed a well-polarized epithelial morphology similar to that in mature hepatocytes [12]. Expression of OSM was restricted in CD45$^+$ hematopoietic cells, while OSMR was

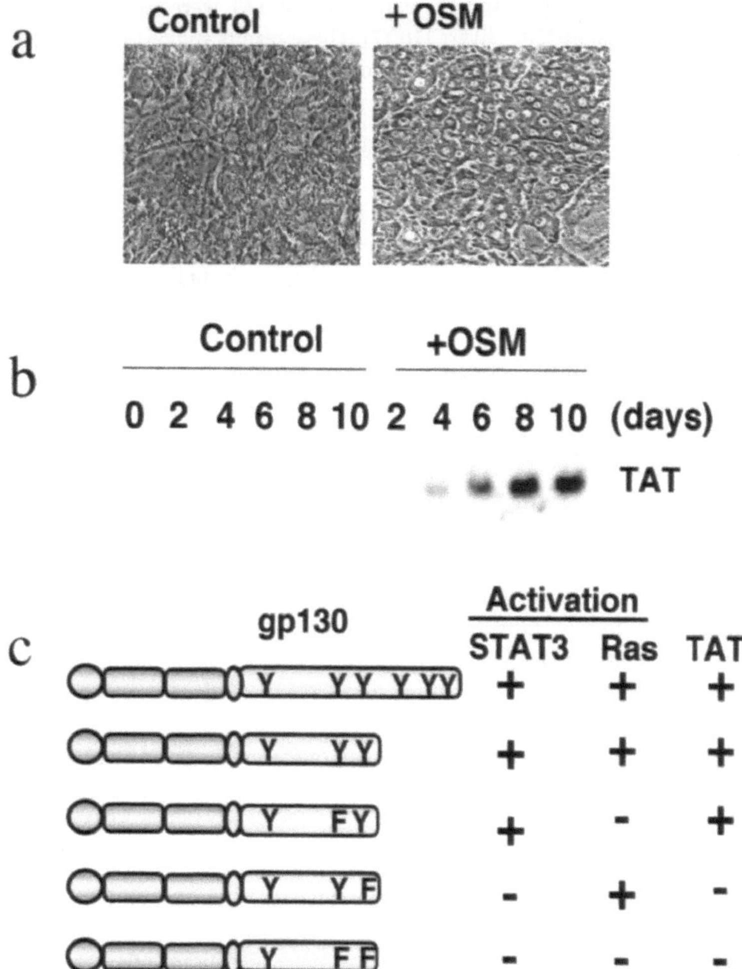

Fig. 1a–c. Oncostatin M (OSM) promotes differentiation of fetal hepatocytes in vitro. **a** Phase-contrast images of cultured fetal hepatocytes in the absence (*control*) or presence of (*+OSM*) of OSM at 10 ng/ml in combination with 10^{-7} M dexamethasone. **b** Expression of a hepatic differentiation marker gene by OSM. The expression of tyrosine amino transferase (*TAT*) was examined by Northern blot analysis. **c** Mutant forms of gp130 were retrovirally introduced into fetal hepatocytes and their ability to induce expression of TAT was examined. Y indicates tyrosine residue in gp130 and F shows the substitution of tyrosine to phenylalanine. The ability of the mutants to activate Ras and STAT3 (signal transducer and activator of transcription protein 3) is also shown

expressed in fetal hepatocytes, suggesting that OSM is a paracrine factor produced in hematopoietic cells that act on neighboring hepatocytes.

Although gp130 knockout (gp130$^{-/-}$) mice of the C57/BL6 genetic background die around E14, gp130$^{-/-}$ mice of the ICR genetic background often survive until birth, allowing us to analyze late fetal liver development [10]. Primary cultures of fetal hepatocytes prepared from gp130$^{-/-}$ mice failed to respond to OSM stimulation [17]. The accumulation of glycogen and the expression of TAT were significantly reduced in peri- and neonatal gp130$^{-/-}$ livers [10,17]. These results suggest that OSM-gp130 signaling is important for embryonic liver development in vitro and in vivo.

Functional Maturation of Fetal Hepatocytes is Dependent on STAT3

It is well known that the Jak-STAT and Ras pathways are activated by OSM in various cell types [1]. In fetal hepatocyte cultures, Jak1, STAT3, STAT5, SHP-2, Shc, p70S6 kinase, and mitogen-activated protein kinase were activated by stimulation with OSM [11]. To elucidate the kinds of signaling molecules responsible for the induction of fetal hepatocyte differentiation, we constructed retroviral vectors with a cDNA encoding a mutant form of the signaling molecules downstream of gp130; e.g., dominant-negative forms of STAT3 (ΔSTAT3), STAT5 (ΔSTAT5), Ras (RasN17), and SHP-2 (C463A), or an active form of Ras (RasV12). Expression of these mutant forms of signaling molecules made it possible to analyze the signaling pathways responsible for the OSM-induced differentiation of fetal hepatocytes. Among these molecules, ΔSTAT3, but not ΔSTAT5, strongly suppressed the differentiation of fetal hepatocytes induced by OSM (Fig. 1c). The gene expression of differentiation markers (*TAT* and *G6Pase*) and the synthesis of glycogen induced by OSM, were inhibited by ΔSTAT3. Interestingly, morphological maturation induced by OSM, as described above, was not affected by ΔSTAT3. Therefore, the functional maturation of fetal hepatocytes induced by OSM is dependent on STAT3, but the morphological maturation is independent of STAT3. However, it should be noted that fetal hepatocytes differentiated without the activation of STAT3 when they were cultured at a high cell density, suggesting the presence of an alternative pathway for the differentiation of fetal hepatocytes in vitro [17].

Morphological Maturation of Fetal Hepatocytes is Dependent on K-Ras

Adherence junctions (AJs) are one of the types of intercellular architecture that connect adjacent cells, and E-cadherin-based AJs are typical in epithelial tissues such as liver [18]. In the absence of OSM, E-cadherin was distributed in a diffuse pattern throughout the cell membrane; however, it localized to AJs, and tight cell-cell contact was formed in response to OSM. Retrovirus-mediated expression of a dominant negative form of Ras, RasN17, completely abolished the formation of AJs induced by OSM. These results suggest that OSM induced the formation of AJs through the Ras pathway.

There are three classical Ras family proteins, H-Ras, N-Ras, and K-Ras. It was reported that knockout mice deficient in both H-Ras and N-Ras developed normally [19], whereas K-Ras$^{-/-}$ mice died at around E15 and exhibited abnormalities of various organs, including liver [20]. In our primary culture system, rapid activation of K-Ras was induced in response to OSM. These results imply that K-Ras is involved in the formation of AJs induced by OSM. The gene expression of differentiation markers (*G6Pase* and *TAT*) was induced by OSM in primary cultures of fetal hepatocytes derived from K-Ras$^{-/-}$, N-Ras$^{-/-}$, and H-Ras$^{-/-}$ mice, as well as the double-knockout of H-Ras and N-Ras, indicating that all these Ras-knockout fetal hepatocytes have potential to response to OSM. However, the translocation of E-cadherin to AJs induced by

OSM was abolished in K-Ras$^{-/-}$ fetal hepatocytes. Retrovirus-mediated K-Ras gene transfer into K-Ras$^{-/-}$ fetal hepatocytes rescued the formation of E-cadherin-based AJs in response to OSM. These results indicate that K-Ras specifically mediates OSM-induced signaling for the formation of AJs in fetal hepatocytes.

Terminal Differentiation of Fetal Hepatocytes is Induced by Extracellular Matrices and OSM

As described above, fetal hepatocytes derived from E14 mouse embryo acquire various functions, such as the expression of G6Pase and TAT, synthesis of glycogen, and clearance of ammonia, in response to OSM in vitro. However, the expression of adult-liver specific enzymes such as TO and several cytochrome p450s was not induced by OSM [10,17,21], indicating that some other factor(s) must be required for the terminal differentiation of hepatocytes. There are many reports that primary cultures of adult hepatocytes rapidly lose certain liver-specific functions such as the expression of P450s, albumin, and α1-antitrypsin. However, the ECM derived from Engelbreth-Holm-Swarm mouse sarcoma (EHS) gel is known to maintain the expression of liver-specific genes in cultured adult hepatocytes. These results suggest that ECM regulates the terminal differentiation of hepatocytes. We therefore examined the effects of EHS gel in combination with OSM on parameters of terminal differentiation, such as the expression of TO and P450s in fetal hepatocytes in vitro. After 5 days' cultivation of fetal hepatocytes in the presence of OSM, EHS gel was added to the culture medium and an additional 2 days' cultivation was performed. The expression of TO, as well as that of P450 genes (*P450-2B10*, *P450-cb*), was induced in this culture system. The enzymatic activity of P450 was also enhanced by EHS gel in combination with OSM [21]. These results suggest that the terminal differentiation of fetal hepatocytes derived from E14 embryo is induced by EHS gel in combination with OSM. Importantly, expression of the *TO* gene was not induced by EHS gel alone, suggesting that serial treatment of the cells with EHS gel following stimulation with OSM is essential for the terminal differentiation of fetal hepatocytes. Thus, we are now able to reproduce the developmental processes of liver from the mid-fetal to the adult stage in vitro by using OSM and EHS gel (Fig. 2).

Role of OSM in Liver Regeneration

The promotion of differentiation of fetal hepatocytes by OSM in vitro, and the liver defects observed in gp130$^{-/-}$ mice, suggest that OSM plays an important role in liver development in vivo. Recently, we generated OSMR$^{-/-}$ mice to investigate the role of OSM in vivo; however, the mice developed normally and no apparent liver defects were observed. This result suggests that the functions of OSM are compensated by other cytokines of the IL-6 family in liver development in vivo. It has been shown, by using IL-6$^{-/-}$ mice, that IL-6 is important for the initial step of liver regeneration [15,16]. Because OSM is a member of the IL-6 family of cytokines, we investigated the involvement of OSM in liver regeneration. Although OSM and OSMR were barely detectable in normal liver, the expression of both mRNAs was rapidly upregulated in response to liver injury induced by CCl$_4$ and partial hepatectomy. CCl$_4$-induced liver

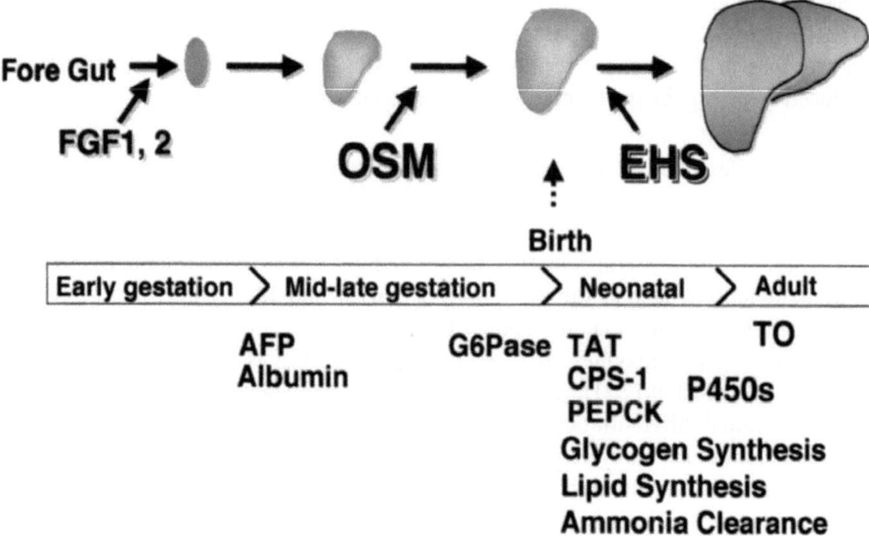

Fig. 2. Process of liver development. Hepatic progenitor cells arise from foregut endodermal cells in response to fibroblast growth factor (*FGF*)-1,2 derived from neighboring cardiac mesoderm to form a liver bud at embryonic days 8–9 (E8–9). Then committed hepatoblasts proceed through several stages of maturation during development. Primary culture of fetal hepatocytes derived from E14 embryo reproduced this stepwise maturation process in the presence of OSM and Engelbreth-Holm-Swarm mouse sarcoma (*EHS*) gel. Fetal hepatocytes treated with OSM expressed genes for peri/neonatal hepatocyte markers, such as *G6Pase*, *TAT*, and phosphoenolpyruvate carboxykinase (*PEPCK*), and acquired various metabolic functions, as mentioned in the Fig. Treatment of the cells with EHS gel followed by OSM induced the gene expression of terminal differentiation markers such as tryptophan oxygenase (*TO*) and cytochrome P450 species (*P450s*). *AFP*, alpha-fetoprotein; *CPS-1*, carbamoyl phosphatase synthetase-1

injury, as evidenced by centrilobular necrosis and increased levels of alanine aminotransferase (ALT) and aspartate aminotransferase (AST) in serum, was enhanced in OSMR$^{-/-}$ mice compared with wild-type mice. In OSMR$^{-/-}$ livers after CCl$_4$-injury, activation of STAT3 was strongly suppressed, and the number of proliferating-cell nuclear antigen (PCNA)-positive hepatocytes was approximately 20% of that in the wild-type liver. Consistent with PCNA staining, the expression of cyclin D1, which is induced in the G$_1$ phase and promotes G$_1$/S transition in the cell cycle, was also decreased in OSMR$^{-/-}$ livers. The restoration of liver mass after hepatectomy was also delayed in OSMR$^{-/-}$ mice. These results strongly suggest that OSMR-mediated signaling plays an important role in the initiation of hepatocyte proliferation in liver regeneration.

Remodeling of the ECM during liver regeneration is important for reconstitution of the liver architecture and is strictly regulated by matrix metalloproteinases (MMPs) and tissue inhibitors of matrix metalloproteinases (TIMPs) [22]. Several investigators reported that expression of TIMP-1 was upregulated by OSM in vitro and in vivo [23,24]. In wild-type livers, expression of the *TIMP-1* gene was undetectable before injury and was strongly induced at 48 h after injury. In contrast, expression of *TIMP-1* after injury was strongly suppressed, to an almost undetectable level, in OSMR$^{-/-}$ livers. These results suggest that OSM is a major regulator of TIMP-1 during liver injury.

The phenotypes observed in OSMR$^{-/-}$ mice are quite similar to those that have been shown in IL-6$^{-/-}$ mice [15,16]. Because both OSM and IL-6 are cytokines that share the gp130 receptor subunit as a common signal transducer and are produced in Kupffer cells in response to injury, there may be redundancy between OSM and IL-6 in liver. However, as the disruption of either one of these cytokine genes resulted in a similar phenotype, an important question remains as to the relationship between IL-6 and OSM. Double-knockout of the *IL-6* and *OSMR* genes may answer this question.

Conclusion

We have shown, using an in vitro culture system and knockout mice, that OSM and the OSM receptor (OSMR/gp130) play an important role in liver development and regeneration. Besides OSM, there are several factors that regulate both liver development and liver regeneration. For example, HGF, which was originally identified by its activity to stimulate liver regeneration, is also important for embryonic liver development. Both HGF$^{-/-}$ mice and c-Met$^{-/-}$ mice die in the embryonic stage and show liver defects [25–27]. Nuclear factor κB (NFκB), a transcription factor activated by TNF-α, also plays a crucial role in both liver development and liver regeneration. Knockout of a subunit of NFκB (RelA) resulted in the massive apoptosis of hepatocytes and liver dysplasia, leading to embryonic lethality at around E15 in mice [28]. Activation of NFκB by TNF-α is also important for the prevention of hepatocyte apoptosis and the induction of IL-6 expression in liver regeneration [15]. Furthermore, recent studies have revealed many common characteristics between embryonic hepatoblasts (or hepatic stem cells) and oval cells, which are considered to be adult hepatic stem cells. An understanding of the molecular basis of the developmental as well as the regenerative processes in the liver will help us to advance liver regenerative medicine in the future.

Acknowledgments. We are grateful to the members of the Stem Cell Regulation Project of the Kanagawa Academy of Science and Technology for their helpful discussions and sharing of their results. This work was supported in part by Grants-in-Aid for Scientific Research and by the Special Coordination Fund for Promoting Science and Technology from the Ministry of Education, Culture, Sports, Science, and Technology; by a research grant from the Ministry of Health, Labour, and Welfare, the Japan Government; and by CREST, Japan Science and Technology Corporation.

References

1. Miyajima A, Kinoshita T, Tanaka M, Kamiya A, Mukouyama Y, Hara T (2000) Role of oncostatin M in hematopoiesis and liver development. Cytokine Growth Factor Rev 11:177–183
2. Tanaka M, Hara T, Copeland NG, Gilbert DJ, Jenkins NA, Miyajima A (1999) Reconstitution of the functional mouse oncostatin M (OSM) receptor: molecular cloning of the mouse OSM receptor beta subunit. Blood 93:804–815

3. Mukouyama Y, Hara T, Xu M, Tamura K, Donovan PJ, Kim H, Kogo H, Tsuji K, Nakahata T, Miyajima A (1998) In vitro expansion of murine multipotential hematopoietic progenitors from the embryonic aorta-gonad-mesonephros region. Immunity 8:105–114

4. Hara T, Tamura K, de Miguel MP, Mukouyama Y, Kim H, Kogo H, Donovan PJ, Miyajima A (1998) Distinct roles of oncostatin M and leukemia inhibitory factor in the development of primordial germ cells and sertoli cells in mice. Dev Biol 201:144–153

5. Jung J, Zheng M, Goldfarb M, Zaret KS (1999) Regulatory phases of early liver development: paradigms of organogenesis. Nat Rev Genet 3:499–512

6. Orkin SH (1996) Development of the hematopoietic system. Curr Opin Genet Dev 6:597–602

7. Greengard O (1970) The developmental formation of enzymes in rat liver. In: Litwack G (ed) Biochemical actions of hormones. Academic, New York, pp 53–87

8. Haber BA, Chin S, Chuang E, Buikhuisen W, Naji A, Taub R (1995) High levels of glucose-6-phosphatase gene and protein expression reflect an adaptive response in proliferating liver and diabetes. J Clin Invest 95:832–841

9. Nagao M, Nakamura T, Ichihara A (1986) Developmental control of gene expression of tryptophan 2,3-dioxygenase in neonatal rat liver. Biochim Biophys Acta 867:179–186

10. Kamiya A, Kinoshita T, Ito Y, Matsui T, Morikawa Y, Senva E, Nakashima K, Taga T, Yoshida K, Kishimoto T, Miyajima A (1999) Fetal liver development requires a paracrine action of oncostatin M through the gp130 signal transducer. EMBO J 18:2127–2136

11. Ito Y, Matsui T, Kamiya A, Kinoshita T, Miyajima A (2000) Retroviral gene transfer of signaling molecules into murine fetal hepatocytes defines distinct roles for the STAT3 and ras pathways during hepatic development. Hepatology 32:1370–1376

12. Matsui T, Kinoshita T, Morikawa Y, Tohya K, Katsuki M, Ito Y, Kamiya A, Miyajima A (2002) K-Ras mediates cytokine-induced formation of E-cadherin-based adherens junctions during liver development. EMBO J 21:1021–1030

13. Michalopoulos GK, DeFrances MC (1997) Liver regeneration. Science 276:60–66

14. Fausto N, Laird AD, Webber EM (1995) Liver regeneration. 2. Role of growth factors and cytokines in hepatic regeneration. FASEB J 9:1527–1536

15. Cressman DE, Greenbaum LE, DeAngelis RA, Ciliberto G, Furth EE, Poli V, Taub R (1996) Liver failure and defective hepatocyte regeneration in interleukin-6-deficient mice. Science 274:1379–1383

16. Kovalovich K, DeAngelis RA, Li W, Furth EE, Ciliberto G, Taub R (2000) Increased toxin-induced liver injury and fibrosis in interleukin-6-deficient mice. Hepatology 31:149–159

17. Kojima N, Kinoshita T, Kamiya A, Nakamura K, Nakashima K, Taga T, Miyajima A (2000) Cell density-dependent regulation of hepatic development by a gp130-independent pathway. Biochem Biophys Res Commun 277:152–158

18. Gumbiner BM (1996) Cell adhesion: the molecular basis of tissue architecture and morphogenesis. Cell 84:345–357

19. Umanoff M, Edelmann W, Pellicer A, Kucherlapti R (1995) The murine N-ras is not essential for growth and development. Proc Natl Acad Sci USA 92:1709–1713

20. Koera K, Nakamura K, Nakao K, Miyoshi J, Toyoshima K, Hatta T, Otani H, Aiba A, Katsuki M (1997) K-Ras is essential for the development of the mouse embryo. Oncogene 15:1151–1159

21. Kamiya A, Kojima N, Kinoshita T, Sakai Y, Miyajima A (2002) Maturation of fetal hepatocytes in vitro by extracellular matrices and oncostatin M: induction of tryptophan oxygenase. Hepatology 35:1351–1359

22. Knittel T, Mehde M, Grundmann A, Saile B, Scharf JG, Ramadori G (2000) Expression of matrix metalloproteinases and their inhibitors during hepatic tissue repair in the rat. Histochem Cell Biol 113:443–453

23. Richards CD, Kerr C, Tanaka M, Hara T, Miyajima A, Pennica D, Botelho F, Langdon CM (1997) Regulation of tissue inhibitor of metalloproteinase-1 in fibroblasts and acute phase proteins in hepatocytes in vitro by mouse oncostatin M, cardiotrophin-1, and IL-6. J Immunol 159:2431–2437
24. Kerr C, Langdon C, Graham F, Gauldie J, Hara T, Richards CD (1999) Adenovirus vector expressing mouse oncostatin M induces acute-phase proteins and TIMP-1 expression in vivo in mice. J Interferon Cytokine Res: 1195–1205
25. Schmidt C, Bladt S, Goedecke S, Brinkmann V, Zschiesche W, Sharpe E, Gherardi E, Birchmeier C (1995) Scatter factor/hepatocyte growth factor is essential for liver development. Nature 373:699–702
26. Uehara Y, Mori C, Noda T, Shiota K, Kitamura N (1995) Placental defect and embryonic lethality in mice lacking hepatocyte growth factor/scatter factor. Nature 373: 702–705
27. Bladt F, Riethmacher D, Isenmann S, Aguzzi A, Birchmeier C (1995) Essential role for the c-met receptor in the migration of myogenic precursor cells into the limb bud. Nature 376:768–771
28. Beg AA, Sha WC, Bronson RT, Ghosh S, Baltimore D (1995) Embryonic lethality and liver degeneration in mice lacking the RelA component of NF-kappaB. Nature 376: 167–170

Hepatocyte Growth Factor Accelerates Proliferation of Hepatic Oval Cells in a 2-Acetylaminofluorene/Partial Hepatectomy Model in the Rat

Akio Ido[1,2], Satoru Hasuike[1], Hirofumi Uto[1], Akihiro Moriuchi[1,2], and Hirohito Tsubouchi[1,2]

Summary. In the rat, oval cells are thought to be hepatic stem-cell candidates. In humans, oval-like cells are also present in injured liver tissue, and are thought to play an important role in liver regeneration. The proliferation of oval cells in the liver in a 2-acetylaminofluorene/partial hepatectomy model in the rat was stimulated by treatment with hepatocyte growth factor (HGF), a major agent promoting the proliferation of mature hepatocytes. In the rat liver, periportal basophilic areas, consisting of oval cells, were significantly larger in rats treated with HGF than in those without HGF on day 7. Expressions of α-fetoprotein (AFP) and c-Kit were detected in the oval cells by immunohistochemistry. Enhanced expression of c-Met was also observed in the oval cells in comparison with the findings in surrounding mature hepatocytes; and tyrosine phosphorylation of c-Met in liver tissues was increased at 7 days of treatment with HGF. These results indicate that HGF promotes the proliferation of both mature hepatocytes and hepatic progenitor cells, and plays an important role in the regeneration of injured liver.

Key words. Hepatocyte growth factor, Oval cell, Liver regeneration, 2-Acetylaminofluorene, Partial hepatectomy

Introduction

Adult mammalian liver has been shown to have a high regenerative capacity. In rodents, loss of liver mass of up to two-thirds produced by surgical or chemical means induces the normal regenerative process [1]. However, when 2-acetylaminofluorene (2-AAF) is continuously administered to such animals, the process is slowed, due to the lack of epithelial cell division; and a new source of cells, called oval cells, appear to help with repair of the liver. Oval cells are considered to play an important role in hepatic growth and development [2–4]. Furthermore, hepatic oval cells are capable of differentiation into several lineages, including hepatocytes and bile duct cells [5–7]. While it has been shown that hepatic oval cells play a part in the regeneration of severely damaged liver, the mechanisms by which the oval cells accomplish liver regeneration are poorly understood.

[1]Second Department of Internal Medicine, Miyazaki Medical College, 5200 Kihara, Kiyotake, Miyazaki 880-1692, Japan
[2]Department of Experimental Therapeutics, Translational Research Center, Kyoto University Hospital, 54 Shogoin-Kawahara-cho, Sakyo-ku, Kyoto 606-8507, Japan

Hepatocyte growth factor (HGF), originally purified from the plasma of patients with fulminant hepatic failure, is one of the major agents promoting the proliferation of mature hepatocytes [8,9]. It also shows mitogenic, motogenic, and morphogenic activities in a wide variety of cells that express the HGF receptor, c-Met, which is a transmembrane protein that possesses an intracellular tyrosine kinase domain [10,11]. Moreover, HGF has been shown to play an essential role in the regeneration of liver, as well as in its development [1,12,13]. In this study, we examined the effect of HGF on the proliferation of oval cells in a 2-AAF/two-thirds partial hepatectomy (PH) model in the rat.

Rat Model of 2-AAF/PH and HGF Administration

Six-week-old male Fisher rats were given 2-AAF (150 mg/day) daily for 5 days, and then a two-thirds partial hepatectomy was performed (day 0) (Fig. 1). Recombinant human HGF was given for 7 days by osmotic pumps implanted in the peritoneal cavity on day 0. In this rat model, levels of serum human HGF increased significantly after the implantation of the osmotic pumps, and continued to increase during 7 days of HGF treatment. An increase in HGF content and an increase in the tyrosine phosphorylation of the HGF receptor, c-Met, in liver tissues were also observed on day 8 of HGF administration. These results indicate that the increased serum human HGF that was released from the osmotic pumps functioned through c-Met tyrosine phosphorylation in liver tissues.

c-Met is Strongly Expressed in Oval Cells, and HGF Accelerates the Proliferation of Hepatic Oval Cells

To examine the effect of HGF administration on the expression of c-Met and the proliferation of oval cells, liver tissues were obtained before and after partial hepatectomy (days 0, 4, 8, and 12). c-Met expression was immunohistochemically stimulated in oval

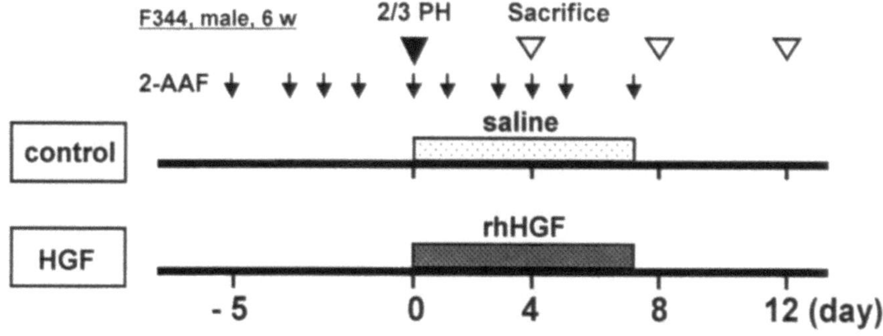

Fig. 1. Six-week-old (*6 w*) male Fisher rats were given 2-acetylaminofluorene (*2-AAF*; 150 mg/day) daily for 5 days, and then a two-thirds partial hepatectomy (*PH*) was performed (*day 0*). Recombinant human hepatocyte growth factor (*HGF*) (*rhHGF*; 200 μg/day) or saline (*control*) was given for 7 days by osmotic pumps implanted in the peritoneal cavity on day 0

Table 1. Summary of immunohistochemical analysis

	Day		
	4	8	12
c-Met	±	3+	2+
HGF (+)	±	3+	2+
AFP	±	2+	2+
HGF (+)	+	2+	±
c-Kit	+	2+	+
HGF (+)	+	3+	+
CK8	±	2+	3+
HGF (+)	±	2+	+
CK18	±	2+	3+
HGF (+)	±	2+	2+

AFP, α-fetoprotein; HGF, hepatocyte growth factor; CK, cytokeratin

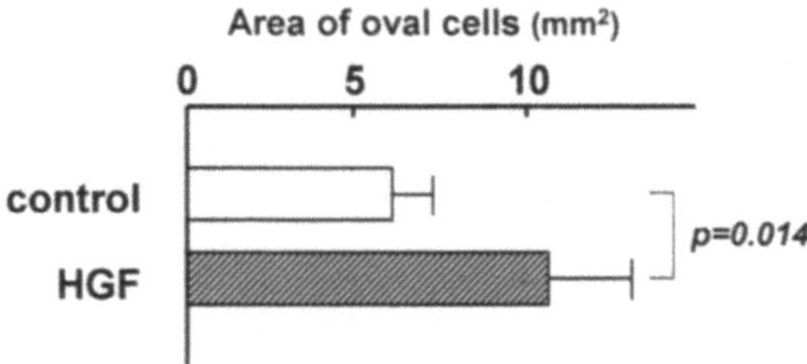

Fig. 2. Effect of HGF on oval-cell proliferation. Liver tissue specimens were stained with hematoxiylin-eosin, and the areas of oval cells measured. Results are shown as the sum of all of the areas in three fields of liver tissue specimens ($n = 4$). Total areas of oval-cell clusters were significantly enlarged in HGF-treated animals on day 7

cells, in comparison with the findings in surrounding mature hepatocytes, while HGF administration did not affect c-Met expression (Table 1). On the other hand, the areas of oval cell compartments were enlarged by HGF administration, and periportal basophilic areas, consisting of oval cells, were significantly larger in rats treated with HGF than in those without HGF on day 7 ($P = 0.014$; Fig. 2). These results indicate that HGF treatment stimulated the proliferation of oval cells.

Effect of HGF on the Expression of α-Fetoprotein (AFP), c-Kit, Cytokeratin (CK)8, and CK18

We immunohistochemically examined the expressions of AFP, c-Kit, CK8, and CK18 (Table 1). In rats treated with HGF, the expression of AFP was detected on day 4, increased on day 8, and declined on day 12, whereas AFP-positive cells appeared on day 8 in control animals. Although the expression of c-Kit was observed in oval cells, regardless of HGF treatment, the number of c-Kit-positive cells increased on day 8 in animals treated with HGF. The expression of CK8 and CK18 in bile duct epithelial cells was more apparent than that in hepatocytes in normal liver tissues. In the 2-AAF/PH rat model, enhanced CK8 expression was observed in oval cells, and this was decreased by HGF administration on day 12. CK18 expression, which was also enhanced in oval cells, was not affected by HGF treatment. These results indicated that HGF might affect not only the proliferation but also the differentiation of oval cells.

Conclusion

Treatment with HGF induced the proliferation of oval cells in the liver of a 2-AAF/PH rat model. These results indicated that HGF promotes the proliferation of both mature hepatocytes and hepatic progenitor cells, and plays an important role in the regeneration of injured livers. Although further investigation is necessary to clarify the involvement of HGF in the differentiation as well as in the proliferation of oval cells, our findings suggest that the administration of HGF could become a new treatment modality to induce liver regeneration in patients with liver failure, or in adult recipients having living-related partial liver transplantations.

References

1. Michalopoulos GK, DeFrances MC (1997) Liver regeneration. Science 276:60–66
2. Farber E (1956) Similarities in the sequence of early histologic changes induced in the liver of the rat by ethionine, 2-acetylaminofluorene, and 3′-methyl-4-dimethylaminoazobenzene. Cancer Res 16:142–151
3. Evarts RP, Nagy R, Marsden E, Thorgeirsson SS (1987) A precursor product relationship exists between oval cells and hepatocytes in rat liver. Carcinogenesis 8:1737–1740
4. Farber E (1991) Hepatocyte proliferation in stepwise development of experimental liver cell cancer. Dig Dis Sci 36:973–978
5. Thorgeirsson SS (1993) Hepatic stem cells. Am J Pathol 142:1331–1333
6. Fausto N (1990) Oval cells and liver carcinogenesis: an analysis of cell lineages in hepatic tumors using oncogene transfection techniques. Prog Clin Biol Res 331: 325–334
7. Signal SH, Brill S, Reid LM (1992) The liver as a stem cell and lineage system. Am J Physiol 263:G139–G148
8. Gohda E, Tsubouchi H, Nakayama H, Hirono S, Takahashi K, Koura M, Hashimoto S, Daikuhara Y (1986) Human hepatocyte growth factor in plasma from patients with fulminant hepatic failure. Exp Cell Res 166:139–150
9. Gohda E, Tsubouchi H, Nakayama H, Hirono S, Sakiyama O, Takahashi K, Miyazaki H, Hashimoto S, Daikuhara Y (1998) Purification and partial characterization of hepatocyte growth factor from plasma of a patient with fulminant hepatic failure. J Clin Invest 81:414–419
10. Rubin JS, Bottaro DP, Aaronson SA (1993) Hepatocyte growth factor/scatter factor and its receptor, the c-met proto-oncogene product. Biochim Biophys Acta 1155: 357–371

11. Zarnegar R, Michalopoulos GK (1995) The many faces of hepatocyte growth factor: from hepatopoiesis to hematopoiesis. J Cell Biol 129:1177–1180
12. Boros P, Miller CM (1995) Hepatocyte growth factor: a multifunctional cytokine. Lancet 345:293–295
13. Scimidt C, Bladt F, Goedecke S, Brinkmann V, Zschiesche W, Sharpe M, Gherardi E, Birchmeier C (1995) Scatter factor/hepatocyte growth factor is essential for liver development. Nature 373:699–702

Stem Cells and Liver Repopulation: Current Reality and Prospects for the Future

David A. Shafritz

Summary. Stem cells can be derived either from growing embryos or from certain somatic tissues with continuous proliferative activity and high turnover, such as bone marrow hematopoietic cells and epithelial cells of the intestinal mucosa and skin. Whether such cells exist in other tissues and organs has been controversial for many years, but recent studies have clearly identified cells with stem-cell properties in muscle, brain, liver, and pancreas. This Chapter will review the general characteristics of stem cells, the evidence for progenitor or stem cells in the liver, the liver-cell transplantation models in which such cells have been studied, the differentiation of cells of hematopoietic and other origin into hepatocytes after transplantation into the liver, and liver repopulation by transplanted cells.

Key words. Stem Cells, Plasticity, Liver regeneration, Cell transplantation, Liver repopulation

General Properties of Stem Cells

The properties of stem cells have been defined based on studies of tissues that show continuous turnover and self-renewal, such as the bone marrow and intestinal epithelium [1,2]. Stem cells are generally considered to exhibit four major characteristics: (1) self-renewal or maintenance (do not proliferate rapidly and are slowly cycling); (2) multipotency (capable of producing progeny in at least two lineages); (3) longterm tissue repopulation after their transplantation; and (4) serial transplantability. Progenitor cells are the progeny of stem cells. In contrast to stem cells, progenitor cells are generally rapidly dividing, but, nonetheless, they are capable of only short-term tissue repopulation. Progenitor cells may be multipotent or unipotent, but also, in contrast to stem cells, they are not self-renewing or capable of serial transplantation. Fully differentiated, organ- or tissue-specific somatic cells in adult mammalian tissues are generally considered to be nonproliferative, with one important exception, the hepatocyte (see later sections of this chapter).

Marion Bessin Liver Research Center, Albert Einstein College of Medicine, 1300 Morris Park Avenue, Bronx, NY 10461, U.S.A.

Stem Cells During Liver Development

Classical embryological studies have traced the proliferation and differentiation of stem cells into hepatocytes and bile duct epithelial cells during normal liver development [3–6]. On embryonal day (ED) 8.5 in the mouse, undifferentiated endodermal cells of the ventral foregut migrate into the septum transversum, where they come into contact with mesenchymal cells and begin to express α-fetoprotein (AFP) at ED 9.0, a process referred to as determination or specification [7]. This is followed by albumin expression at around ED 9.5. The morphology of the cells then changes to that of the hepatoblast (an early progenitor cell). Hepatoblasts proliferate rapidly between ED12 and ED16 and are bipotent, subsequently diverging along two distinct lineages, the hepatocyte and the cholangiocyte, beginning just prior to ED16, a process referred to as commitment [8]. After ED16, the cells progress along one or the other of these lineages and no longer retain their bipotential properties, although they continue to proliferate (so-called late or "committed" progenitor cells). The bile ducts and hepatic cords begin to form at this time, and this process continues until 1–2 weeks after birth, at which time maturation of the liver structure is completed [9].

Evidence for Hepatocyte Progenitor Cells

The existence of progenitor or stem cells in the adult liver was postulated more than 40 years ago by Wilson and Leduc [10], based on studies in rodents, in which small epithelial cells in the distal cholangioles of the bile ducts appeared to be responsible for restoration of the liver mass after dietary injury. Subsequently, Farber [11] identified a population of small undifferentiated epithelial cells emanating from the portal region after treatment of rats with carcinogens, such as 2-acetylaminofluorine (2-AAF), which he termed "oval" cells. He did not believe that these cells were hepatic progenitor cells [12], but Thorgeirsson and coworkers (Evarts et al. [13,14]) showed that liver "oval" cells induced to proliferate by 2-AAF differentiated into hepatocytes after two-thirds partial hepatectomy (PH). During this process, many known hematopoietic stem cell genes, such as *c-Kit*, *CD-34*, *flt3 receptor*, and *LIF*, are activated, further suggesting that oval cells have stem-cell-like properties, i.e., they are facultative stem cells (for review, see reference 15). Oval cells can also be activated by treating rats with D-galactosamine, a noncarcinogenic agent that causes extensive liver injury and hepatic necrosis, but also blocks proliferation of hepatocytes, as does 2-AAF. In the D-galactosamine model, the specific transition from an undifferentiated oval cell into a fully differentiated hepatocyte has been demonstrated by both molecular in situ hybridization and immunohistochemical methods [16]. In these studies, our laboratory and that of Nelson Fausto have identified AFP-positive oval cells in the normal liver [16,17], providing further evidence that early progenitor or stem-like cells are present in the adult liver. These cells are in a quiescent state and can be activated by either 2-AAF/PH or D-galactosamine injury to produce oval cells, which can subsequently differentiate into hepatocytes.

Liver Regeneration and Hepatic Cell Transplantation

The ability of the liver to regenerate is unique among solid organs in mammalian species. During normal liver regeneration following PH, mature hepatocytes undergo one or two rounds of cell division to restore the liver mass [18]. However, the oval cell compartment is not activated under these circumstances. If adult hepatocytes are transplanted into the liver in conjunction with PH, they too will proliferate through one or two cell divisions. From these studies, it was concluded that although hepatocytes can divide and restore liver mass, they are terminally differentiated and have very limited proliferative capacity. However, studies over the past decade have completely revolutionized our thinking concerning both the proliferative capacity of differentiated hepatocytes and also what controls the phenotype of hepatic and other somatic cells (plasticity).

Model Systems for Liver Repopulation by Transplanted Hepatocytes

In the early 1990s, Sangren et al. [19] developed a transgenic mouse model to study protease function by inserting the urokinase plasminogen activator gene (*uPA*) into the liver under control of the albumin promoter. In alb-uPA transgenic mice, most of the uPA was secreted into the bloodstream, where it was being studied as a thrombolytic agent. However, some of the protease remained in the liver, causing severe inflammation and extensive necrosis, and most animals died. However, some animals survived, and, in those animals, large clusters of normal liver cells were observed, sometimes replacing almost the entire liver. The normal cells had deleted the *uPA* transgene, an event which occurred with a frequency of 1×10^{-5}–1×10^{-6}. These cells proliferated extensively in response to continuous liver injury and had an enormous selection advantage for survival compared to host hepatocytes still expressing the toxic *uPA* transgene. Isolated, single-cell suspensions of genetically marked normal hepatocytes were then transplanted into *uPA* transgenic mice and these cells also repopulated the liver [20]. In this model, it was calculated that, during liver repopulation, each transplanted hepatocyte underwent around 12–14 divisions, dispelling the widely held concept that mature hepatocytes have only limited proliferative capacity.

A second model for liver repopulation, the fumarylacetate hydrolase (FAH) null mouse, was subsequently developed by Grompe and coworkers (Overturf et al. [21]) to study the human disorder, hereditary tyrosinemia type 1 (HT1). In this model, tyrosine metabolism is blocked at the last step in tyrosine catabolism, the conversion of fumarylacetoacetate to fumarate, acetoacetate, and succinate. This leads to the accumulation of upstream metabolic intermediates in tyrosine catabolism that are toxic and cause continuous liver injury, chronic liver disease, cirrhosis, and hepatocellular carcinoma. Similar to results obtained with *uPA* transgenic mice, wild-type (wt) hepatocytes transplanted into FAH null mice repopulated the liver, and restored normal liver architecture and function [21]. In the FAH null model, as few as 10,000 wt hepatocytes can be serially transplanted through seven generations of mice, with total liver repopulation in each mouse [22]. Assuming that all hepatocytes have equal proliferative capacity, it was concluded that hepatocytes have the ability to undergo a minimum of 77 cell divisions. Therefore, the regenerative capacity of fully mature parenchymal cells in the liver is essentially infinite.

In both of these models of liver repopulation, a unique combination of experimental conditions in the host environment permitted massive proliferation of transplanted hepatocytes and replacement of damaged liver tissue: (1) the liver is under a constant state of massive injury/regeneration; and (2) the transplanted cells have an enormous selective advantage for survival compared to host hepatocytes. An alternative strategy to achieve selective repopulation by transplanted cells would be to disrupt the proliferative capacity of host hepatocytes, and then transplant cells with normal proliferative capacity. Our laboratory, in conjunction with Ezio Laconi, developed such a strategy by treating rats with retrorsine, a pyrrolizidine alkaloid that alkylates cellular DNA and prevents hepatocytes from proliferating [23]. Treatment with retrorsine creates a longlasting mito-inhibitory environment in the liver, so that when retrorsine-treated rats are subjected to PH, endogenous hepatocytes are unable to proliferate, but transplanted hepatocytes can respond normally to restore liver mass.

We combined retrorsine/PH treatment with a cell transplantation model in which dipeptidylpeptidase IV (DPPIV)$^+$ hepatocytes are transplanted into the liver of a DPPIV$^-$ mutant rat. The fate and phenotype of the transplanted cells is then determined by enzyme histochemistry to detect DPPIV$^+$ cells in the liver of transplanted animals. Transplanted hepatocytes become fully integrated into the hepatic plates, surprisingly without disturbing or compressing the surrounding parenchyma [23]. The transplanted hepatocytes form hybrid bile canaliculi with endogenous hepatocytes and maintain a normal hepatic parenchymal structure [23]. In this model, up to 99% repopulation of the retrorsine-treated liver can be achieved with adult wt hepatocytes. The liver mass was restored to near normal size and the transplanted cells were fully active biochemically and physiologically [23,24]. The retrorsine model has recently been successfully adapted to mice [25].

Another model to block proliferation of endogenous hepatocytes is irradiation injury, which, when coupled with PH or ischemic liver injury to act as a liver proliferative stimulus, is an excellent model for liver repopulation by transplanted hepatocytes [26,27]. Induction of apoptosis by injecting Fas antibody (Jo2) has also been used in mice to injure the host liver and stimulate proliferation of transplanted hepatocytes containing the anti-apoptotic gene *Bcl-2* [28]. In one variation of this model, many rounds of liver injury by Jo2 antibody, in conjunction with in vivo transduction of hepatocytes with a retrovirus expressing *Bcl-2*, led to 85% replacement of the host liver [29]. Rogler and colleagues (Peterson et al. [30]) developed a mouse model for liver repopulation which can accept xenographs by cross-breeding of uPA transgenic mice to Rag(–/–) mice, which are T- and B-cell-deficient and are thus immunotolerant to transplanted cells across species barriers. In uPA(+/+)/Rag2(–/–) mice, transplanted woodchuck hepatocytes can repopulate the host liver [30]. Human hepatocytes can also proliferate and partially repopulate the liver of uPA(+/+)/Rag(–/–) mice [31]. The SCID/bg mouse, which is even more immunotolerant than the Rag2(–/–) null mouse, has also been cross-bred to the uPA(+/+) transgenic mouse, and this model also accepts human liver cell xenographs [32]. Human hepatocyte-transplanted uPA(+/+)/Rag(–/–) mice have been successfully infected with human hepatitis B virus (HBV) [31] and human hepatocyte-transplanted uPA(+/+)/SCID/bg mice have been infected with hepatitis C virus (HCV) [32], providing new opportunities to study antiviral therapies for HBV and HCV infection in animal systems.

Repopulation of the Liver by Transplanted Fetal Liver Cells

All of the above studies used animal models in which the host liver was markedly perturbed. Our hope was to achieve the same outcome in a normal liver environment, and we reasoned that this might be possible using either activated progenitor cells or liver stem cells. We isolated cell fractions from the liver and pancreas that were enriched for "oval" progenitor cells, in the former case by treating rats with D-galactosamine [16,33] and in the latter case by inducing the proliferation of AFP-positive small epithelial cells in the pancreas in response to pancreatic atrophy secondary to Cu depletion [34,35]. In both cases, the progenitor cells engrafted in the liver and differentiated into mature hepatocytes [33]. However, the hepatocytic clusters produced by the transplanted cells were small, and significant liver repopulation was not observed. We then isolated a similar cell fraction from the rat ED12–14 fetal liver, and transplanted these cells into adult rats that had undergone PH [36]. Under these conditions, we achieved 5%–10% repopulation of the normal liver. Transplanted ED12-14 fetal liver epithelial cells underwent up to nine to ten cell divisions, forming very large clusters. Using double-label immunohistochemistry/in situ hybridization, we demonstrated that transplanted cells were still proliferating 6 months after transplantation. In contrast to studies in transgenic and knockout mice or the retrorsine model in rats, these results were achieved in a normal liver environment in which there was no apparent selection for transplanted cells other than their innate proliferative capacity. Under the same conditions, mature hepatocytes did not proliferate beyond the first month following their transplantation, and there was no significant liver repopulation [36]. With fetal liver epithelial cells, most of the liver repopulation occurred between 2 and 6 months following transplantation, long after the liver had returned to normal size following two-thirds PH. The majority of the proliferating cell clusters contained both hepatocytes and bile ducts, suggesting bipotency of cells producing these clusters. At 4 and 6 months post-ED14 fetal liver cell transplantation, we also noted secondary or satellite clusters containing both hepatocytes and bile duct structures, and these clusters also increased in size over time. In our more recent studies, we have found that liver repopulation by transplanted fetal liver cells continues for up to 1 year, and by using larger numbers of transplanted cells (40–50 × 10^6 unfractionated rat ED14 fetal liver cells), we have been able to obtain 30%–35% repopulation of the whole normal adult liver, with repopulation exceeding 50% in many areas (our unpublished observations). With cells isolated from ED16 or ED18 fetal livers (post-commitment), we see a few scattered small clusters of hepatocytes or rudimentary bile duct structures, but no significant repopulation of the normal adult rat liver. These studies demonstrated that "precommitment" or early fetal liver epithelial cells transplanted into the normal adult rat liver exhibit three major properties of stem cells; namely, bipotency, proliferation for an extended period, and longterm tissue repopulation [36]. Because we have not yet demonstrated serial transplantability of fetal liver cells, we refer to the repopulating cells as fetal liver stem/progenitor cells [36].

Plasticity and the Role of the Tissue Microenvironment

As is evident from recent studies in brain, bone marrow, liver, and pancreas, somatic cells exhibit considerable flexibility in their gene expression properties, and cells derived from one organ can differentiate into cells of another organ after their engraftment into the latter site. This property is referred to as plasticity. Perhaps the most spectacular observation regarding plasticity is the finding that a cell line derived from rat liver epithelial cells (WB344) can differentiate into other tissue-specific phenotypes when transplanted into other organs, including myocytes when transplanted into the heart, hematopoietic cells in the bone marrow, and glandular epithelium in the prostate [37,38]. However, a word of caution is in order, because the whole concept of plasticity has been challenged by recent studies reporting fusion between hematopoietic cells or brain cells and embryonic stem cells in culture with subsequent differentiation into many different somatic phenotypes [39,40].

Liver Repopulation by Hematopoietic Stem Cells

In most innovative studies, Petersen et al. [41] and Theise et al. [42] transplanted either crude bone marrow or purified hematopoietic stem cells into lethally irradiated rats and mice, respectively, and in both instances, donor-derived cells with the morphologic appearance of hepatocytes were identified in the liver. Liver repopulation in these systems was estimated to be around 0.1% by Petersen and 1%–2% by Theise. Lagasse et al. [43] conducted similar studies with purified hematopoietic stem cells in FAH null mice and, in this case, repopulation was up to 30% at 6 months, and the liver exhibited normal metabolic function. However, in FAH null mice, most recent studies have determined that most of the repopulating cells represent fusions between transplanted hematopoietic cells and host hepatocytes [44,45]. Under these conditions, the transplanted wild-type bone marrow cells provide the missing *FAH* gene, which allows the hepatocytic fusion partner to proliferate massively in the toxically injured liver environment [44,45].

In human studies conducted by Theise et al. [46] and Alison et al. [47], the presence of Y chromosome-positive hepatocytes has been found in the liver of female recipients of male bone marrow cells and in male recipients of orthotopic liver transplants from female donors. The presence of donor-derived bile duct cells has also been reported [46] and in this study, estimates of liver repopulation by hematopoietic cells were as high as 35%–40%.

In other studies in mice [48], donor-derived epithelial cells have been identified in multiple organs, including the lung, liver, gastrointestinal tract, and hair follicles, after transplantation of a single hematopoietic stem cell into sublethally irradiated animals. Similar findings have been found in humans following bone marrow transplantation, and the longer the bone marrow recipient survived the greater the repopulation of specific organs [49]. Verfaillie and coworkers (Schwartz et al. [50]) have established mesenchymal stem cell lines from the adult rodent and human bone marrow, termed multipotent adult progenitor cells (MAPC). Under specialized growth conditions in culture, including the use of matrigel, fibroblast growth *factor* (FGF)-4 and hepatocyte growth factor (HGF), these cells differentiate into hepatocyte-like cells [50]. When

MAPC are transplanted into appropriate hosts, they differentiate into multiple organ lineages, including lung, liver, and gut, in addition to hematopoietic cells [51]. The implications of these and the above findings are enormous in terms of their potential for liver reconstitution, correction of genetic diseases, and treatment of other disorders associated with abnormal liver function.

Other Recently Described Systems to Study Liver Repopulation by Transplanted Cells

Several recent studies have reported that human hematopoietic stem cells (HSC) isolated from either the bone marrow or umbilical cord blood can differentiate in the liver of NOD/Scid mice into cells exhibiting a hepatocytic phenotype and expressing liver-specific genes [52–54]. The frequency of these cells is very low (less than 1/1000 or 1/10,000), but liver injury seems to increase their number. The cells engraft in the liver, using normal homing mechanisms for hematopoietic cells involving SDF-1 and CXCR4 interaction, and both the metalloproteinase MMP-9 and HGF appear to augment liver engraftment [54]. At present, however, fusion between hematopoietic cells and host hepatocytes has not been identified for human HSC expressing a hepatocytic phenotype in the NOD/Scid mouse liver [55]. Another hematopoietic cell transplantation model in mice, using the GFP marker gene for donor cells, has also been developed recently (see chapter by Terai et al. in this volume) and shows promise as an animal model system to study liver repopulation by transplanted hematopoietic cells.

Conclusions

Innovative studies during the past decade have shown that both hepatocytes and hematopoietic stem cells can repopulate the liver under highly selective conditions of severe continuous liver injury or disruption of endogenous hepatocyte proliferation. In addition, fetal liver stem/progenitor cells can do this in a normal liver environment, and it appears that fetal cells (or more primitive stem cells) have a greater proliferative and repopulation potential than differentiated somatic cells. It has also been observed that cells migrating through the circulation or transplanted into a secondary organ can differentiate into a specific somatic phenotype in the host organ of residence. However, under what conditions this represents plasticity versus fusion between the circulating cells and somatic cells in the host organ into which they have become engrafted, remains to be determined. Regardless of the mechanism, the transplanted cells become physically and physiologically incorporated into normal parenchymal structures and appear to function normally, at least in the liver. These observations suggest that tissue restoration by cell transplantation may become a practical reality in the near future.

Acknowledgments. The author thanks his colleagues, postdoctoral fellows, and students who conducted the various studies reported from his laboratory, and the many scientists who have made outstanding contributions to this area of research. Research supported in part by NIH grants RO1-DK17609, RO1 DK56496, and P30-DK41296.

References

1. Pierce GB, Shikes R, Fink LM (1978) Cancer: a problem of developmental biology. Prentice Hall, Englewood Cliffs NJ, pp 1–242
2. Potten CS, Loeffler M (1990) Stem cells: attributes, cycles, spirals, pitfalls and uncertainties: lessons for and from the crypt. Development 110:1101–1120
3. DuBois AM (1963) The embryonic liver. In: Rouiller CH (ed) The liver. New York, Academic
4. Wilson JW, Groat CS, Leduc EH (1963) Histogenesis of the liver. Ann NY Acad Sci 111: 8–22
5. Le Douarin NM (1975) An experimental analysis of liver development. Med Biol 53: 427–455
6. Houssaint E (1980) Differentiation of mouse hepatic primordium: an analysis of tissue interactions in hepatocyte differentiation. Cell Growth Differ 9:269–279
7. Zaret K (2000) Liver specification and early morphogenesis. Mech Dev 92:83–88
8. Marceau N, Blouin M-J, Noel M, Torok N, Loranger A (1992) The role of biopotential progenitor cells in liver ontogenesis and neoplasia. In: Sirica AE (ed) The role of cell types in hepatocarcinogenesis. CRC, Boca Raton, FL, pp 121–149
9. Van Eyken R, Sciot R, Desmet V (1988) Intrahepatic bile duct development in the rat: a cytokeratin-immunohistochemical study. Lab Invest 59:52–59
10. Wilson JW, Leduc EH (1958) Role of cholangioles in restoration of the liver of the mouse after dietary injury. J Pathol Bacteriol 76:441–449
11. Farber E (1956) Similarities of the sequence of the early histological changes induced in the liver of the rat by ethionine, 2-acetylaminofluorene, and 3′-methyl-4-dimethylaminoazobenzene. Cancer Res 16:142–148
12. Tatematsu M, Ho RH, Kaku T, Ekem JK, Farber E (1984) Studies on the proliferation and fate of oval cells in the liver of rats treated with 2-acetylaminofluorine and partial hepatectomy. Am J Pathol 114:418–430
13. Evarts RP, Nagy P, Marsden E, Thorgeirsson SS (1987) A precursor-product relationship exists between oval cells and hepatocytes in rat liver. Carcinogenesis 8:1737–1740
14. Evarts RP, Nagy P, Nakatsukasa H, Marsden E, Thorgeirsson SS (1989) In vivo differentiation of rat liver oval cells into hepatocytes. Cancer Res 49:1541–1547
15. Grisham JW, Thorgeirsson SS (1997) Liver stem cells. In: Potten CS (ed) Stem cells. London, Academic, pp 233–282
16. Dabeva MD, Shafritz DA (1993) Activation, proliferation and differentiation of progenitor cells into hepatocytes in the D-galactosamine model of liver regeneration. Am J Pathol 143:1606–1620
17. Lemire JM, Shiojiri N, Fausto N (1991) Oval cell proliferation and the origin of small hepatocytes in liver injury induced by D-galactosamine. Am J Pathol 139: 535–552
18. Michalopoulous GK, DeFrances MC (1997) Liver regeneration. Science 276:60–66
19. Sangren EP, Palmiter RD, Heckel JL, Daugherty CC, Brinster RL, Degan JL (1991) Complete hepatic regeneration after somatic deletion of an albumin-plasminogen activator transgene. Cell 66:245–256
20. Rhim J, Sangren EP, Degan JL, Palmiter RD, Brinster RL (1994) Replacement of diseased mouse liver by hepatic cell transplantation. Science 263:1149–1152
21. Overturf K, Al-Dhalimy M, Tanguay R, Brantly M, Ou CN, Finegold M, Grompe M (1996) Hepatocytes corrected by gene therapy are selected in vivo in a murine model of hereditary tyrosinaemia type 1. Nat Genet 12:226–273
22. Overturf K, Al-Dhalimy M, Ou CN, Finegold M, Grompe M (1997) Serial transplantation reveals the stem-cell like regenerative potential of adult mouse hepatocytes. Am J Pathol 151:1273–1280

23. Laconi E, Oren R, Mukhopadhyay D, Hurston E, Laconi S, Pani P, Dabeva MD, Shafritz DA (1998) Long term, near total liver replacement by transplantation of isolated hepatocytes. Am J Pathol 153:319–329

24. Oren R, Dabeva M, Petkov P, Hurston E, Laconi E, Shafritz DA (1999) Restoration of normal serum albumin levels in Nagase analbuminemic rats using a newly described strategy for hepatocytes transplantation. Hepatology 29:75–81

25. Guo D, Fu T, Nelson JA, Superina RA, Soriano HE (2002) Liver repopulation after cell transplantation in mice treated with retrorsine and carbon tetrachloride. Transplantation 73:1818–1824

26. Guha C, Sharma A, Gupta S, Alfieri A, Gorla GR, Gagandeep S, Sokhi R, Roy-Chowdhury N, Tanaka KE, Vikram B, Roy-Chowdhury J (1999) Amelioration of radiation-induced liver damage in partially hepatectomized rats by hepatocytes transplantation. Cancer Res 59:5871–5874

27. Malhi H, Gorla GR, Irani AN, Annamaneni P, Gupta S (2002) Cell transplantation following oxidative hepatic preconditioning with radiation and ischemia-reperfusion leads to extensive liver repopulation. Proc Natl Acad Sci USA 99:13,114–13,119

28. Mignon A, Guidotti JE, Mitchell C, Farbre M, Wernet A, De La Coste A, Soubrane O, Gilgenkrantz H, Kahn A (1998) Selective repopulation of normal mouse liver by Fas/CD-95 resistant hepatocytes. Nat Med 4:1185–1188

29. Guidotti JE, Mallet VO, Mitchell C, Fabre M, Schoevaert D, Opolon P, Parlier D, Lambert M, Kahn A, Gilgenkrantz H (2001) Selection of in vivo retrovirally transduced hepatocytes leads to efficient and predictable liver repopulation. FASEB J 15:1849–1851

30. Petersen J, Dandri M, Gupta S, Rogler CE (1998) Liver repopulation with xenogenic hepatocytes in B and T cell-deficient mice leads to chronic hepadnavirus infection and clonal growth of hepatocellular carcinoma. Proc Natl Acad Sci USA 95:310–315

31. Dandri M, Burda MR, Torok E, Pollok JM, Iwanska A, Sommer G, Rogiers X, Rogler CE, Gupta S, Will H, Greten H, Petersen J (2001) Repopulation of mouse liver with human hepatocytes and in vivo infection with hepatitis B virus. Hepatology 33:981–988

32. Mercer DF, Schiller DE, Elliott JF, Douglas DN, Hao C, Rinfret A, Addison WR, Fischer KP, Churchill TA, Lakey JR, Tyrrell DL, Kneteman NM (2001) Hepatitis C virus replication in mice with chimeric human livers. Nat Med 7:927–933

33. Dabeva MD, Hwang SG, Vasa SR, Hurston E, Novikoff PM, Hixson DC, Gupta S, Shafritz DA (1997) Differentiation of pancreatic epithelial progenitor cells into hepatocytes following transplantation into rat liver. Proc Natl Acad Sci USA 94:7356–7361

34. Rao MS, Dwivedi RS, Yeldandi AV, Subbarao V, Tan X, Usman MI, Thangada S, Nemali MR, Kumar S, Scarpelli DG (1989) Role of periductal and ductular epithelial cells of the adult rat pancreas in pancreatic hepatocyte lineage. A change in the differentiation commitment. Am J Pathol 134:1069–1086

35. Dabeva MD, Hurston E, Shafritz DA (1995) Transcription factor and liver-specific mRNA expression in facultative progenitor cells of liver and pancreas. Am J Pathol 147:1633–1648

36. Sandhu JS, Petkov PM, Dabeva MD, Shafritz DA (2001) Stem cell properties and repopulation of the rat liver by fetal liver epithelial progenitor cells. Am J Pathol 159:1323–1334

37. Malouf NN, Coleman WB, Grisham JW, Lininger RA, Madden VJ, Sproul M, Anderson PA (2001) Adult-derived stem cells from the liver become myocytes in the heart in vivo. Am J Pathol 158:1929–1935

38. Grisham JW (2001) Plasticity and potency of liver stem-like cells (abstract). Hepatology 34:21A

39. Terada N, Hamazaki T, Oka M, Hoki M, Mastaler DM, Nakano Y, Meyer EM, Morel L, Petersen BE, Scott E (2002) Bone marrow cells adopt the phenotype of other cells by spontaneous cell fusion. Nature 416:542–545

40. Ying QL, Nichols J, Evans EP, Smith AG (2002) Changing potency by spontaneous fusion. Nature 416:545–548

41. Petersen BE, Bowen WC, Patrene KD, Mars WM, Sullivan AK, Murase N, Boggs SS, Greenberger JS, Goff JP (1999) Bone marrow as a potential source of hepatic oval cells. Science 284:1168–1170

42. Theise ND, Badve S, Saxena R, Henegariu O, Sell S, Crawford JM, Krause DS (2000) Derivation of hepatocytes from bone marrow cells in mice after radiation-induced myeloablation. Hepatology 31:235–240

43. Lagasse E, Connors H, Al-Dhalimy M, Reitsma M, Dohse M, Osborne L, Wang X, Finegold M, Weissmann IL, Grompe M (2000) Purified hematopoietic stem cells can differentiate to hepatocytes in vivo. Nat Med 6:1229–1234

44. Wang X, Willenbring H, Akkari Y, Torimaru Y, Foster M, Al-Dhalimy M, Lagasse E, Finegold M, Olson S, Grompe M (2003) Cell fusion is the principal source of bone-marrow-derived hepatocytes. Nature 422:897–901

45. Vassilopoulos G, Wang PR, Russell DW (2003) Transplanted bone marrow regenerates liver by cell fusion. Nature 422:901–904

46. Theise ND, Nimmakayalu M, Gardner R, Illei PB, Morgan G, Teperman L (2000) Liver from bone marrow in humans. Hepatology 32:11–16

47. Alison MR, Poulsom R, Jeffery R, Dhillon AP, Quaglia A, Jacob J, Novelli M, Prentice G, Williamson J, Wright NA (2000) Hepatocytes from non-hepatic adult stem cells. Nature 406:257 (brief communication, only one page)

48. Krause DS, Theise ND, Collector MI, Henegariu O, Hwang S, Gardner R, Neutzel S, Sharkis SJ (2001) Multi-organ, multi-lineage engraftment by a single bone marrow-derived stem cell. Cell 105:369–377

49. Korbling M, Katz RL, Khanna A, Ruifrok AC, Rondon G, Albitar M, Champlin RE, Estrov Z (2002) Hepatocytes and epithelial cells of donor origin in recipients of peripheral-blood stem cells. N Engl J Med 345:738–746

50. Schwartz RE, Reyes M, Koodie L, Jiang Y, Blackstad M, Lund T, Lenvik T, Johnson S, Hu WS, Verfaillie CM (2002) Multipotent adult progenitor cells from bone marrow differentiate into functional hepatocyte-like cells. J Clin Invest 109:1291–1302

51. Jiang Y, Jahagirdar BN, Reinhardt RL, Schwartz RE, Keene CD, Ortiz-Gonzalez XR, Reyes M, Lenvik T, Lund T, Blackstad M, Du J, Aldrich S, Lisberg A, Low WC, Largaespada DA, Verfaillie CM (2002) Pluripotency of mesenchymal stem cells derived from adult marrow. Nature 418:41–49

52. Danet GH, Luongo JL, Butler G, Lu MM, Tenner AJ, Simon MC, Bonnet DA (2002) C1qR$_p$ defines a new human stem cell population with hematopoietic and hepatic potential. Proc Natl Acad Sci USA 99:10,441–10,445

53. Wang X, Ge S, McNamara G, Hao Q-L, Crooks GM, Nolta JA (2003) Albumin-expressing hepatocyte-like cells develop in the livers of immune-deficient mice that received transplants of highly purified human hematopoietic stem cells. Blood 101:4201–4208

54. Kollet O, Shivtiel S, Chen YQ, Suriawinata J, Thung SN, Dabeva MD, Kahn J, Spiegel A, Dar A, Samira S, Goichberg P, Kalinkovich A, Arenzana-Seisdedos F, Nagler A, Hardan I, Revel M, Shafritz DA, Lapidot T (2003) HGF, SDF-1, and MMP-9 are involved in stress-induced human CD34+ stem cell recruitment to the liver. J Clin Invest 112:160–169

55. Newsome PN, Johannessen I, Boyle S, Samuel K, Rae F, Forrester L, Turner ML, Hayes PC, Harrison D, Bickmore W, Plevris JN (2002) Human cord-blood derived cells can differentiate into hepatocytes in the NOD SCID mouse liver with no evidence of cellular fusion (abstract). Hepatology 36:212 (no. 181)

Strategy for the Development of Cell Therapy Using Bone Marrow Cells to Repair Damaged Liver

SHUJI TERAI, ISAO SAKAIDA, NAOKI YAMAMOTO, KAORU OMORI, and KIWAMU OKITA

Summary. Recently, the plasticity of stem cells in bone marrow to differentiate into other cell lineages has been reported. If we can use stem cells in bone marrow, we can easily isolate hepatic stem cells to regenerate liver. In particular, cell therapy using autologous bone marrow cells to regenerate blood vessels has already been done clinically. To develop cell therapy using bone marrow cells to repair damaged liver, we have to understand the mechanism by which bone marrow cells differentiate into hepatocytes. In this chapter, we report a strategy for the development of cell therapy for liver regeneration.

Key words. Bone marrow cell, Stem cell, Cell therapy, Liver regeneration

Introduction

Although liver transplantation is an established therapy for fulminant hepatitis and other severe liver diseases, the scarcity of brain-dead donors, particularly in Japan, limits the use of transplantation [1]. Regenerative medicine using stem cells will be an attractive therapy for patients suffering from severe liver failure. Regenerative medicine can be divided into three approaches. One approach is cell therapy, using special cells which have plasticity, such as embryonic stem (ES) cells and tissue-specific adult stem cells [2–4]. A second approach is therapy using tissue engineering techniques [5,6]. The third approach is therapy using bioartifical devices (Fig. 1) [7]. Among these three approaches, we would like to develop a new cell therapy using autologous bone marrow cells (BMCs) to repair damaged liver. Compared with other tissue-specific stem cells, the isolation of stem cells from bone marrow is easier than that of other tissue-specific stem cells [3,8–11]. Cell therapy using autologous BMCs presents few ethical problems and will have many medical applications for treating severe liver, pancreatic, and intestinal disease.

Department of Molecular Science and Applied Medicine (Gastroenterology and Hepatology), Yamaguchi University School of Medicine, 1-1-1 Minami-Kogushi, Ube, Yamaguchi 755-8505, Japan

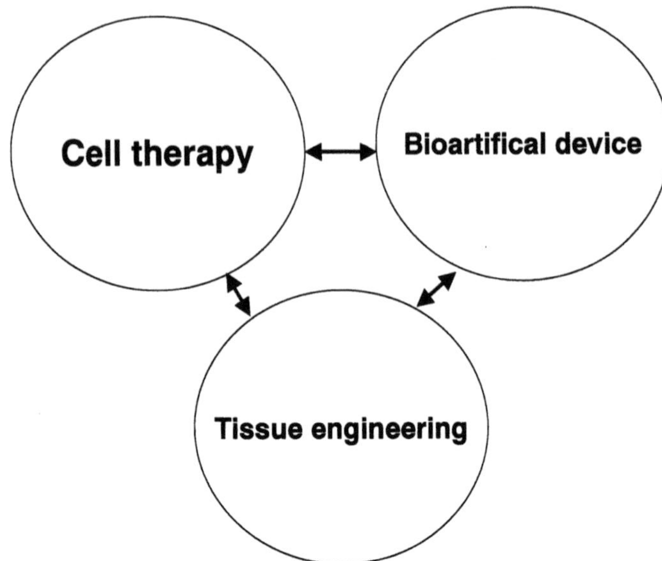

Fig. 1. Approaches to regenerative medicine

Hepatic Stem Cells are Present in Bone Marrow

Peterson et al. [8] and Theise et al. [12] showed the existence of hepatic stem cells in bone marrow by transplanting BMCs from male rats into females, then analyzing the recipients' hepatocytes for Y chromosome markers by fluorescent in situ hybridization (FISH). In human studies, the transdifferentiation of BMCs into hepatocytes was demonstrated by detection of the presence of Y chromosome markers in autopsied liver specimens from male-to-female bone marrow transplant recipients [9,13]. These results show the possibility of new cell therapy using BMCs [14]. On the other hand, after reports that spontaneous cell fusion is an important mechanism for the transdifferentiation of BMCs and tissue-specific stem cells, many people cannot accept the existence of cells in adult BMC that have multipotenty capacity for differentiation [15,16]. Although Laggase et al. [17], using a fumarylacetate hydrolase (FAH)-deficient model, reported that purified hematopoietic stem cells could become transdifferentiated into hepatocytes and compensate liver function, recently they reported that the mechanism of transdifferentiation of BMCs into hepatocytes arose from cell fusion between the BMCs and hepatocytes. Wagers et al. [18] also reported that there was little evidence of plasticity of adult hematopoietic stem cells. In a human study, Tran et al. [19] reported that cell fusion was a rare event, by analyzing for Y chromosome makers, using a FISH technique, in buccal epithelial cells after male-to-female BMC transplantation. On the other hand, Schwarz et al. [20] and Jiang et al. [21] established multipotent adult progenitor cells (MAPCs) in bone marrow with a culture system; these cells were derived from mesenchymal stem cells. At present, the mechanism for the plasticity of (BMCs) is unknown. Moreover, although there are various kinds of cells in bone marrow, we could not confirm which of the cells in bone marrow are the real hepatic stem cells. To develop effective cell therapy with BMCs, we need a better understanding of the regulatory mechanisms that control BMC plasticity and BMC transdifferentiation into nonhematopoietic cell lineages.

Inflammation Signals and Liver Development

Hepatic stem cells can differentiate into hepatocytes under several different conditions [22]. For example, induction of liver damage in rats with 2-acetylaminofluorene and partial hepatectomy (AAF/PH) is one model system for the differentiation of hepatic stem (oval) cells [23]. Some inflammation signals, such as tumor necrosis factor (TNF)-alpha and the nuclear factor (NF)-κB pathway, are crucial for liver regeneration and hepatogenesis, as shown in studies of knockout mice [24–26]. These signals might also regulate the commitment of BMCs to a hepatocyte lineage. If inflammation signals have an important role in the differentiation of BMCs and hepatocytes, we have to analyze the interaction between these signals and the cells. The inflammation signal might create a specific microenvironment "niche" which regulates the differentiation and proliferation of cells [26] (Fig. 2).

Green Fluorescence Protein (GFP)/CCl4 Model: New in vivo Model to Monitor the Transdifferentiation of BMCs into Hepatocytes

To analyze the mechanism of the transdifferentiation of BMCs, we developed a new in vivo model, different from the FAH model, to monitor the differentiation of BMCs into functional hepatocytes [27]. In this model, we transplanted BMCs without adding prior culture. For the liver cirrhosis model in the recipient, we selected a model produced by the injection of carbon tetrachloride (CCl4), carried out for 4 weeks; this model is similar to liver cirrhosis in humans. In this study we used transgenic mice expressing GFP as a source of BMCs to explore the process of differentiation into

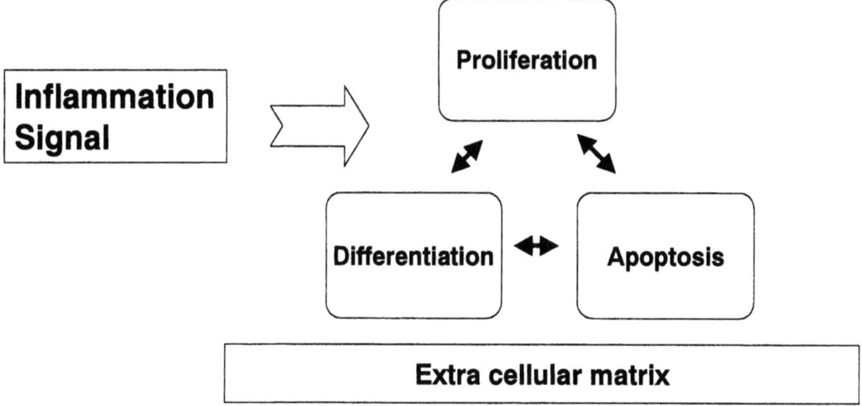

Fig. 2. Differentiation "niche"

hepatocytes [28]. We isolated GFP-positive BMCs and transplanted these GFP-positive BMCs into mice with liver cirrhosis. Mice with liver cirrhosis induced by CCl4 were injected with 1×10^5 nontreated GFP-positive BMCs via the tail vein. In these mice, the transplanted GFP-positive BMCs efficiently migrated into the periportal area of liver lobules after 1 day, and had repopulated one-fourth of the recipient liver by 4 weeks under conditions of persistent liver damage [27]. In contrast, no GFP-positive BMCs were detected following transplantation into control mice with undamaged livers. The BMCs transdifferentiated into functional mature hepatocytes via immature hepatoblasts. Serum albumin was significantly elevated by BMC transplantation to compensate for chronic liver failure. In our model, the transdifferentiation of BMCs into hepatocytes occurred under the conditions of persistent liver damage. These results suggested that the inflammation signal was also important for the transdifferentiation of BMCs into hepatocyte. Inflammation signals such as TNF-alpha and the NF-κB pathway are crucial for liver regeneration and hepatogenesis, as shown in studies of knockout mice [24–26]. The differentiation processes in BMC transdifferentiation and liver development are similar.

Discussion

The result with the GFP/CCl4 model showed that the condition of the recipient and the microenvironment are key factors for successful cell therapy using BMCs. If we consider the use of cell therapy with BMCs to repair damaged liver, we must evaluate the condition of the recipient. If the condition of the recipient is adequate for the transdifferentiation of BMCs into hepatocytes, we will succeed in repairing the damaged liver. To analyze the regulatory mechanism of the transdifferentiation system, our GFP/CCl4 model will be useful. Based on the analysis of this model, we will be able to evaluate the mechanism of transdifferentiation, using the analysis of gene expression and proteomics. By analyzing the mechanism, we will be able to develop a new cell therapy using BMCs to repair damaged liver.

References

1. Terai S, Yamaoto N, Omori K, Sakaida I, Okita K (2002) A new cell therapy using bone marrow cells to repair damaged liver. J Gastroenterol 37(Suppl XIV):162–163
2. Thomson JA, Odorico JS (2002) Human embryonic stem cell and embryonic germ cell lines. Trends Biotechnol 18:53–57
3. Pittenger MF, Mackay AM, Beck SC, Jaiswal RK, Douglas R, Mosca JD, Moorman MA, Simonetti DW, Craig S, Marshak DR (1999) Multilineage potential of adult human mesenchymal stem cells. Science 284:143–147
4. Poulsom R, Alison MR, Forbes SJ, Wright NA (2002) Adult stem cell plasticity. J Pathol 197:441–456
5. Tabata II (2000) The importance of drug delivery systems in tissue engineering 3:80–89
6. Komuro H, Nakamura T, Kaneko M, Nakanishi Y, Shimizu Y (2002) Application of collagen sponge scaffold to muscular defects of the esophagus: an experimental study in piglets. J Pediatr Surg 37:1409–1413

7. Khalili TM, Navarro A, Ting P, Kamohara Y, Arkadopoulos N, Solomon BA, Demetriou AA, Rozga J (2001) Bioartificial liver treatment prolongs survival and lowers intracranial pressure in pigs with fulminant hepatic failure. Artif Organs 25:566–570

8. Petersen BE, Bowen WC, Patrene KD, Mars WM, Sullivan AK, Murase N, Boggs SS, Greenberger JS, Goff JP (1999) Bone marrow as a potential source of hepatic oval cells. Science 284:1168–1170

9. Theise ND, Nimmakayalu M, Gardner R, Illei PB, Morgan G, Teperman L, Henegariu O, Krause DS (2000) Liver from bone marrow in humans. Hepatology 32:11–16

10. Gage FH (2000) Mammalian neural stem cells. Science 287:1433–1438

11. Potten CS (1998) Stem cells in gastrointestinal epithelium: numbers, characteristics and death. Philos Trans R Soc Lond Biol 353:821–830

12. Theise ND, Badve S, Saxena R, Henegariu O, Sell S, Crawford JM, Krause DS (2000) Derivation of hepatocytes from bone marrow cells in mice after radiation-induced myeloablation. Hepatology 31:235–240

13. Korbling M, Katz RL, Khanna A, Ruifrok AC, Rondon G, Albitar M, Champlin RE, Estrov Z (2002) Hepatocytes and epithelial cells of donor origin in recipients of peripheral-blood stem cells. N Engl J Med 346:738–746

14. Orlic D, Kajstura J, Chimenti S, Jakoniuk I, Anderson SM, Li B, Pickel J, McKay R, Nadal-Ginard B, Bodine DM, Leri A, Anversa P (2001) Bone marrow cells regenerate infarcted myocardium. Nature 410:701–705

15. Ying QL, Nichols J, Evans EP, Smith AG (2002) Changing potency by spontaneous fusion. Nature 416:545–548

16. Terada N, Hamazaki T, Oka M, Hoki M, Mastalerz DM, Nakano Y, Meyer EM, Morel L, Petersen BE, Scott EW (2002) Bone marrow cells adopt the phenotype of other cells by spontaneous cell fusion. Nature 416:542–545

17. Lagasse E, Connors H, Al-Dhalimy M, Reitsma M, Dohse M, Osborne L, Wang X, Finegold M, Weissman IL, Grompe M (2000) Purified hematopoietic stem cells can differentiate into hepatocytes in vivo. Nat Med 6:1229–1234

18. Wagers AJ, Sherwood RI, Christensen JL, Weissman IL (2002) Little evidence for developmental plasticity of adult hematopoietic stem cells. Science 297:2256–2259

19. Tran SD, Pillemer SR, Dutra A, Barrett AJ, Brownstein MJ, Key S, Pak E, Leakan RA, Kingman A, Yamada KM, Baum BJ, Mezey E (2003) Differentiation of human bone marrow-derived cells into buccal epithelial cells in vivo: a molecular analytical study. Lancet 361:1084–1088

20. Schwartz RE, Reyes M, Koodie L, Jiang Y, Blackstad M, Lund T, Lenvik T, Johnson S, Hu WS, Verfaillie CM (2002) Multipotent adult progenitor cells from bone marrow differentiate into functional hepatocyte-like cells. J Clin Invest 109:1291–1302

21. Jiang Y, Jahagirdar BN, Reinhardt RL, Schwartz RE, Keene CD, Ortiz-Gonzalez XR, Reyes M, Lenvik T, Lund T, Blackstad M, Du J, Aldrich S, Lisberg A, Low WC, Largaespada DA, Verfaillie CM (2002) Pluripotency of mesenchymal stem cells derived from adult marrow. Nature 418:41–49

22. Grisham JW, Thorgeirsson SS (1997) Liver stem cells. Academic Press, Manchester

23. Golding M, Sarraf CE, Lalani EN, Anilkumar TV, Edwards RJ, Nagy P, Thorgeirsson SS, Alison MR (1995) Oval cell differentiation into hepatocytes in the acetylaminofluorene-treated regenerating rat liver. Hepatology 22:1243–1253

24. Beg AA, Sha WC, Bronson RT, Ghosh S, Baltimore D (1995) Embryonic lethality and liver degeneration in mice lacking the RelA component of NF-kappa B. Nature 376:167–170

25. Li Q, Van Antwerp D, Mercurio F, Lee KF, Verma IM (1999) Severe liver degeneration in mice lacking the IkappaB kinase 2 gene. Science 284:321–325

26. Nishina H, Vaz C, Billia P, Nghiem M, Sasaki T, De la Pompa JL, Furlonger K, Paige C, Hui C, Fischer KD, Kishimoto H, Iwatsubo T, Katada T, Woodgett JR, Penninger JM

(1999) Defective liver formation and liver cell apoptosis in mice lacking the stress signaling kinase SEK1/MKK4. Development 126:505–516

27. Terai S, Sakaida I, Yamamoto N, Omori K, Watanabe T, Ohata S, Katada T, Miyamoto K, Shinoda K, Nishina H, Okita K (In press) An in vivo model for monitoring transdifferentiation of bone marrow cells into functional hepatocytes. The Journal of Biochemistry

28. Okabe M, Ikawa M, Kominami K, Nakanishi T, Nishimune Y (1997) "Green mice" as a source of ubiquitous green cells. FEBS Lett 407:313–319

Bcl-xL as a Critical Apoptosis Antagonist in Hepatocytes and Hepatocellular Carcinoma

Tetsuo Takehara and Norio Hayashi

Summary. Bcl-xL, an anti-apoptotic member of the Bcl-2 family, has been generally thought to be involved in the regulation of apoptosis in the liver, because this molecule tends to be upregulated during liver regeneration, as well as in certain types of liver injury. We employed a Cre/loxP conditional knockout model and found that deletion of the *bcl-x* gene resulted in accelerated apoptosis in hepaocytes in vivo, formally proving the critical role of this molecule in maintaining hepatocyte integrity. Furthermore, Bcl-xL may play an important role during hepatocarcinogenesis, because one-third of human hepatocellular carcinoma (HCC) tissues showed increased expression of Bcl-xL and its knockdown by antisense oligonucleotide stimulated apoptosis in hepatoma cells in response to cellular stresses, such as serum starvation, p53 activation, and staurosporine treatment. It was also found that Bcl-xL was post-translationally modified by deamidation in its loop domain in human liver tissues; deamidated Bcl-xL is a major form in normal liver tissues, whereas the level of deamidated Bcl-xL is lower than that of unmodified Bcl-xL in the majority of HCC tissues. As protein deamidation of Bcl-xL leads to a complete "loss of function" of this anti-apoptotic molecule, HCCs may acquire resistance to apoptosis and a survival advantage by suppressing the deamidation, as well as by increasing the expression of Bcl-xL.

Key words. Bcl-xL, Liver, Apoptosis, Deamidation, Cancer

Introduction

The cell death machinery is a well-conserved system from *Caenorhabditis elegans* to vertebrates, consisting of apoptosis sensor, regulator, adapter, and executioner (Fig. 1). *C. elegans* has a unique molecule for each function. In contrast, we vertebrates possess redundant molecules that have similar structures and share similar functions. In the case of inhibitors of apoptosis, we have at least six CED9 homologs belonging to anti-apoptotic members of the Bcl-2 family: Bcl-2, a prototype of this family, Bcl-xL, Mcl-1, Bcl-w, Bfl-1/A1, and Diva/Boo [1]. From this point of view, the issue of which molecules are expressed and are critically important should be determined for each specific cell type in mammals.

Department of Molecular Therapeutics, Osaka University Graduate School of Medicine, 2-2 Yamada-oka, Suita, Osaka 565-0871, Japan

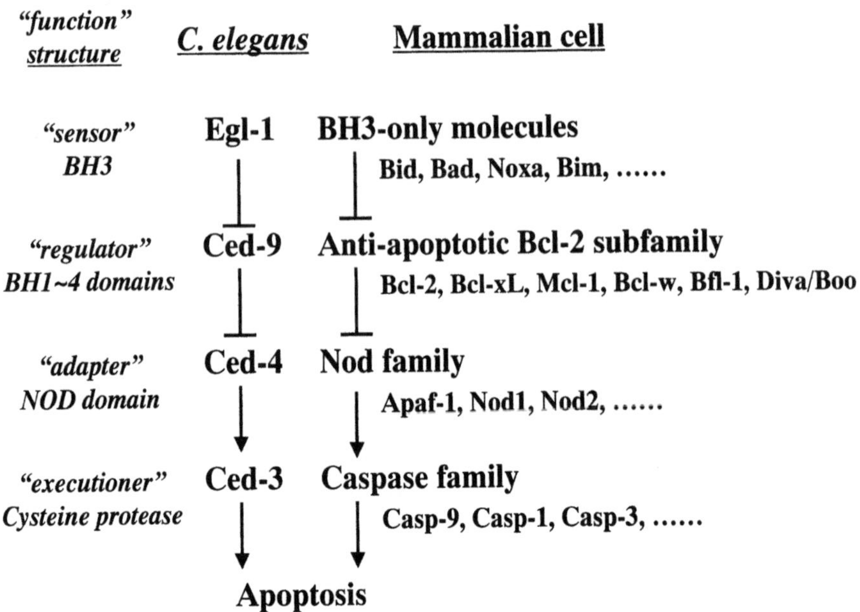

Fig. 1. Comparison of the cell death machinery in *Caenorhabditis elegans* and mammalian cells

Bcl-xL in Hepatocytes

Traditional gene targeting of the anti-apoptotic members of the Bcl-2 family reveals a distinct role for these molecules in developmental and homeostatic processes. Bcl-2 knockout mice are viable but runted and die within a few months of birth from renal failure due to polycystic kidneys [2]. Bcl-w-deficient mice [3,4] and Bfl-1-deficient mice [5] are viable, but show impaired spermatogenesis and accelerated apoptosis in neutrophils, respectively. Diva knockout mice do not show any abnormality, although Diva was shown to be highly expressed in the ovary [6]. Targeted elimination of the *bcl-x* or *mcl-1* gene results in embryonic lethality. A *bcl-x*-deficient embryo dies around embryonic day 13, showing defects in neuronal development and hematopoiesis [7]. The Mcl-1 knockout embryo is the most severe phenotype, not implanting to the uterus [8]. No phenotype in hepatocytes has been reported among these gene-targeted mice.

Hepatocytes express Bcl-xL, Bcl-w, and Mcl-1, but not Bcl-2. Among these molecules, it has been speculated that Bcl-xL may be an important apoptosis regulator in the liver, as this molecule tends to be upregulated in liver regeneration [9,10] and in some types of liver injury [11]. To formally determine the role of Bcl-xL in hepatocytes, we used a Cre-loxP conditional knockout model. When primary cultured hepatocytes isolated from *bcl-x fl/fl* mice were infected with Cre-expressing adenovirus, AdCANCre [12] at a multiplicity of infection (MOI) of 3, the *bcl-x* gene was efficiently deleted and Bcl-xL expression was downregulated to substantially lower levels by 2 days after the infection. The viability of *bcl-x fl/fl* hepatocytes began to decrease 2 days after the infection and reached around 20% on day 3. In contrast, hepatocytes from *bcl-x fl/+* or wild-type littermates did not show any decrease in their viability. The decreased viability of cultured hepatocytes induced by conditional deletion of the *bcl-x* gene was due to increased apoptosis, as evidenced by clear DNA laddering on ethidium bromide-stained agarose gel. To examine the role of Bcl-xL in hepatocytes in vivo, we injected AdCANCre to floxed mice via the tail vein, because adenovirus preferentially infects hepatocytes in vivo. Three days after the injection, more than 80% of the hepatocytes were positive for Cre, based on immunohistochemistry findings and the levels of Bcl-xL were substantially downregulated on Western blot analysis. At this time point, serum alanine aminotransferase (ALT) levels were significantly higher in AdCANCre-injected floxed mice than in the AdCANCre-injected wild-type littermates. TdT-mediated dUTP nick end labeling (TUNEL)-positive hepatocytes were scattered in the livers of AdCANCre-injected fl/fl mice, but could not be detected in the AdCANCre-injected wild-type littermates. These findings provided the first evidence that Bcl-xL expressed in hepatocytes plays an critical role in maintaining the integrity of hepatocytes in vivo, although several anti-apoptotic members of the Bcl-2 family are expressed in hepatocytes.

We have previously demonstrated that Bcl-xL is overexpressed in one-third of human hepatocellular carcinoma (HCC) tissues compared with their noncancerous counterparts, most of which are chronically diseased livers, or normal human liver tissues (Fig. 2) [13]. To determine the role of Bcl-xL expressed in hepatoma cells, we designed an antisense oligonucleotide (ODN) to target the human *bcl-x* translation initiation site, as well as designing three control ODNs, sense, mismatch, and scramble ODNs. When HepG2 cells were transfected with each ODN, the *bcl-x* antisense ODN specifically reduced Bcl-xL expression, but did not produce apoptosis compared with control ODNs. When HepG2 cells were cultured in the presence of 1 µM of staurosporine, a typical apoptosis inducer, *bcl-x* antisense-treated HepG2 cells underwent apoptosis more rapidly than control ODN-treated HepG2 cells. In addition the *bcl-x* antisense-treated HepG2 cells, but not control ODN-treated cells, released cytochrome c into the cytosol upon staurosporine treatment, indicating the disruption of mitochondrial integrity. A similar increase in apoptosis was also found in *bcl-x* antisense-treated HepG2 cells in the absence of serum. Therefore, Bcl-xL endogenously expressed in hepatoma cells is critically important for their survival under cellular stress-inducing conditions.

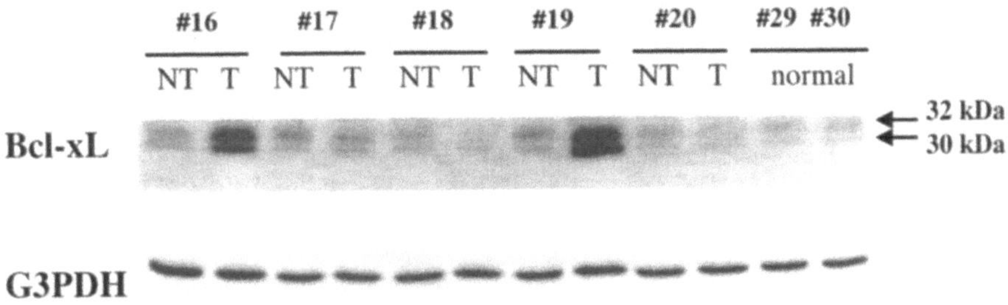

Fig. 2. Bcl-xL in human liver tissues. Expression of Bcl-xL was assessed by Western analysis in pairs of hepatocellular carcinoma (HCC) tissues (*T*), adjacent nontumor liver counterparts (*NT*), and normal livers (*normal*). Bcl-xL migrated as a doublet band of 30 and 32 kDa. Glyceraldehyde-3-phosphate dehydrogenase (*G3PDH*) served as a control for sample loading

p53 and Bcl-xL

p53 is known to play an important role in suppressing tumor development and progression via the transcriptional activation of various genes involved in DNA repair, cell-cycle arrest, and the induction of apoptosis. The *p53* gene is frequently mutated in the advanced stage of HCC, but not in the early phase of HCC. We therefore addressed the issue of whether Bcl-xL expressed in hepatoma cells affects p53-mediated apoptosis. To this end, we transfected Hep3B cells, which are deficient for the *p53* gene, with a temperature-sensitive mutant of *p53*, *p53 Val135*, to establish the 4Bv c lone, which carries the mutant gene, and a control, BT-2E, which only carries the *neo* resistant gene. When the Hep3B 4Bv clone was cultured at 32°C, the *p21* gene, a typical p53 target, was activated. In contrast, culture at 32°C did not affect the expression of *p21* in the Hep3B BT-2E clone, indicating that *p53 Val135* assumes a mutant conformation at 37°C, but a wild-type conformation at 32°C. We transfected the 4Bv and the BT-2E clones with each ODN to modulate Bcl-xL expression and then cultured the cells for 3 days at either 32°C or 37°C. Treatment with the *bcl-x* antisense ODN significantly increased the death of the 4Bv clone at 32°C, but not at 37°C. Importantly, the expression of transcriptionally active p53 at 32°C did not produce cell death in the control ODN-treated 4Bv clone. Cell death was also examined by DNA fragmentation, indicating that the downregulation of Bcl-xL can induce p53-mediated apoptosis. These findings indicate that Bcl-xL endogenously expressed in Hep3B cells blocks p53-mediated apoptosis, implying that overexpression of Bcl-xL may impede p53 tumor suppressor activity in HCC.

Bcl-xL Deamidation

As shown in Fig. 2, Bcl-xL expressed in human liver tissues migrates as a doublet band with molecular masses of approximately 30 and 32 kDa on sodium dodecylsulfate (SDS)-polyacrylamide gel electrophoresis (PAGE). Interestingly, the fast-migrating Bcl-xL (30-kDa band) was expressed at a level higher than that of the slower-migrating Bcl-xL (32-kDa band) in HCC tissues, in contrast to the opposite pattern being shown in nontumor counterparts and normal human livers. The fast-migrating Bcl-xL (30-kDa band) was more abundant than the slower-migrating species (32-kDa band) in hepatoma cell lines, in agreement with the results for HCC tissues. Figure 3 summarizes the ratio of the optical density of the 30-kDa band compared with that of the 32-kDa band (30 kDa/32 kDa). The ratio was greater than 1 in 11 of 20 cases of HCC, in 1 of 20 nontumor tissues, and in none of the 10 normal livers ($P < 0.005$; HCC compared with adjacent nontumor tissue or normal liver by Bonferroni's *t*-test after significant analysis of variance (ANOVA)). Thus, the 32-kDa band is the major form of Bcl-xL in normal and nontumor liver tissues, whereas the density of the 30-kDa band is increased in a majority of HCCs. Based on these observations, we sought to determine the biochemical nature of these two forms of Bcl-xL.

Phosphorylation of Bcl-xL induced by microtuble-disrupting agents and its subsequent slower migration on gel electrophoresis have been described [14]. We tested the hypothesis that the 32-kDa species may be a phosphorylated form of Bcl-xL. A more slowly migrating band at approximately 34 kDa appeared after HepG2 cells were

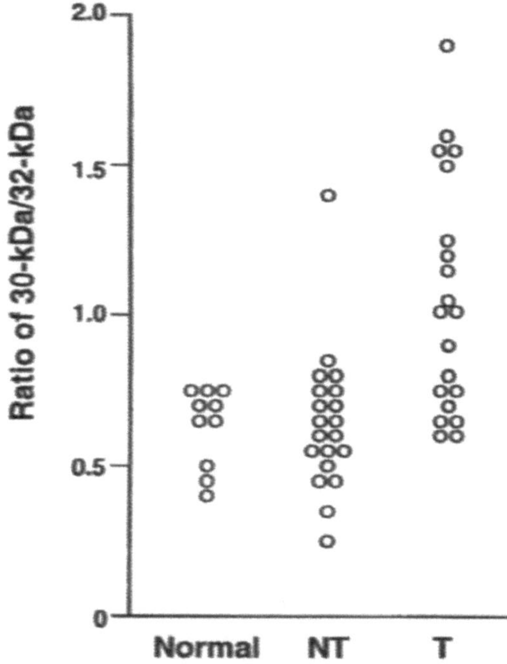

Fig. 3. Differences in Bcl-xL migration on sodium dodecylsulfate-polyacrylamide gel electrophoresis (SDS-PAGE) among human liver tissues. A summary is shown of the ratio of the optical density of the 30-kDa band compared with that of the 32-kDa band (*30-kDa/32-kDa*) in normal livers (*normal*), nontumor livers (*NT*), and HCCs (*T*)

treated with vincristine, a microtuble-disrupting agent. In vitro, λ phosphatase treatment prior to electrophoresis completely abolished this new band, but did not affect the migration pattern of the original two bands. Therefore, the 32-kDa band is not a phosphorylated form of Bcl-xL, as was the case after vincristine treatment.

An asparagine that is followed by a glycine in a polypeptide is susceptible to deamidation, which converts the asparagine residue to a mixture of aspartate and isoaspartate (Fig. 4) [15–17]. Human Bcl-xL contains three asparagine-glycine sequences, at asparagine -52, -66, and -185. Asparagine -52 and -66 are located on the loop domain of Bcl-xL, and asparagine -185 is on the BH2 domain. Therefore, we sought to examine whether the difference in electrophoretic mobility between the 30- and 32-kDa Bcl-xL may have resulted from deamidation of the protein. It is known that alkaline conditions at high temperature augment the rate of deamidation in vitro. We treated HCC tissue lysates with a pH 10 alkaline buffer, and then examined the expression of Bcl-xL by Western blot analysis. Treatment of the tissue lysates with the alkaline buffer for 6 h at 30°C, but not at 4°C, resulted in an increase of the 32-kDa band and a decrease of the 30-kDa band. Treatment of the tissue lysates with the same alkaline buffer for a longer incubation time, 16 h, at the same temperature, further increased the intensity of the 32-kDa band, and caused dissipation of the 30-kDa band. Incubation of the same lysates with a neutral buffer (pH 7.4), at either 4°C or 30°C for 16 h, did not affect the mobility of Bcl-xL on SDS-PAGE. Thus, alkaline conditions, which facilitate protein deamidation, appeared to modify the 30-kDa Bcl-xL and produce the 32-kDa Bcl-xL. To confirm the deamidation of Bcl-xL, we investigated the isoaspartate content of recombinant human Bcl-xL that had been treated with an alkaline buffer, because deamidation converts asparagine residues in polypeptides to a mixture of aspartates

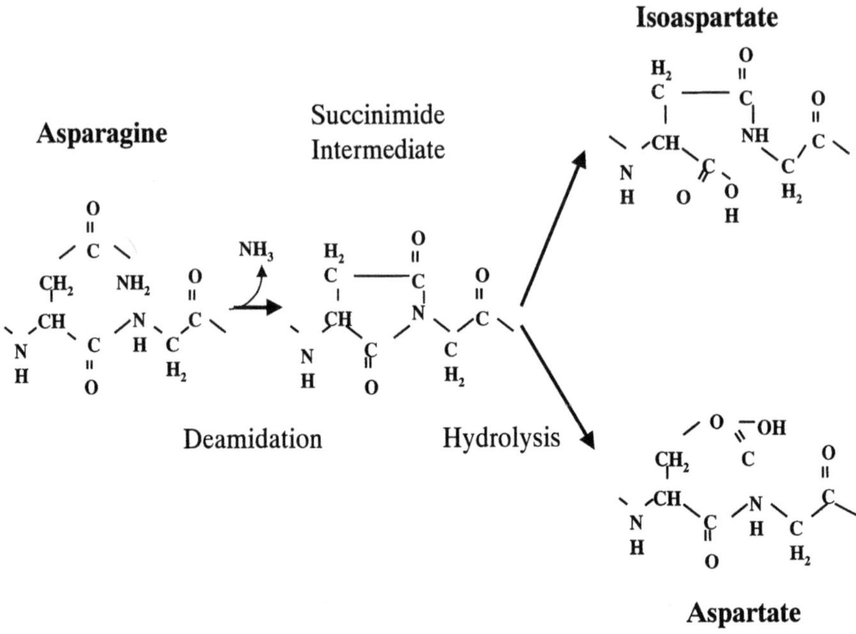

Fig. 4. Asparagine (*Asn*) deamidation. The α-amino of the residue C flanking the Asn makes a nucleophilic attack on the Asn side chain to form a cyclic imide (succinimide) intermediate. This hydrolyzes to a mixture of isoaspartate and aspartate at a ratio of approximately 2:1

and isoaspartates. The methyl-accepting capacity of the recombinant Bcl-xL for protein isoaspartyl methyltransferase, which correlates with the isoaspartate content of the protein, significantly increased after the alkaline treatment. Thus, in vitro alkaline treatment produced deamidation of the Bcl-xL protein and increased its content of isoaspartate, a product of asparagine deamidation. In addition, the same alkaline treatment resulted in a modification of recombinant Bcl-xL that showed slower migration on SDS-PAGE. These results further support the idea that the more slowly migrating species is a deamidated form of the Bcl-xL protein.

Because human Bcl-xL has three candidate sites for asparagine deamidation, we sought to determine which asparagine residues were susceptible to deamidation and responsible for the production of the more slowly migrating Bcl-xL. We prepared seven mutant Bcl-xL constructs, in which alanines were substituted for asparagine -52, -66, or -185. Focus hepatoma cells were transfected with each mutant plasmid, and the migration pattern of Bcl-xL was examined by Western blot. Focus cells that were transfected with a wild-type Bcl-xL expression plasmid expressed Bcl-xL as a doublet band, while a more slowly migrating form of Bcl-xL was not detected in Focus cells that were transfected with an N52A/N66A plasmid. Thus, the substitution of alanines for both asparagine -52 and -66 inhibited the production of the more slowly migrating Bcl-xL. These results indicate that asparagine -52 and -66 residues are the susceptible sites for protein deamidation and that these sites are necessary for the production of the more slowly migrating form of Bcl-xL that was seen on SDS-PAGE (Fig. 5).

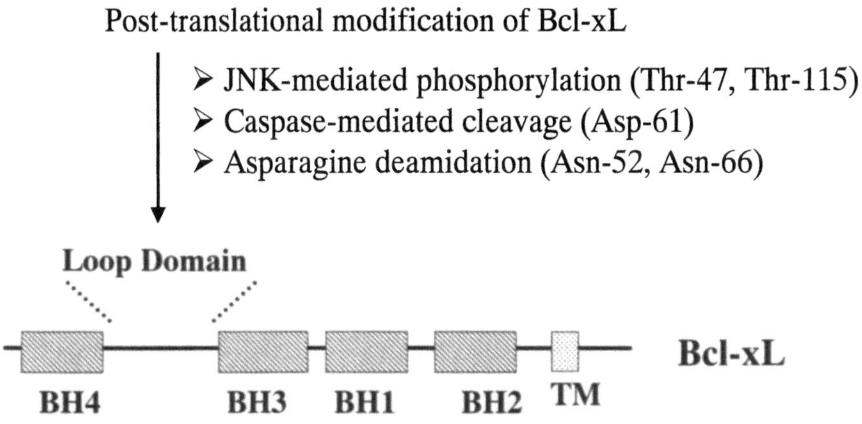

Post-translational modification of Bcl-xL

> ➤ JNK-mediated phosphorylation (Thr-47, Thr-115)
> ➤ Caspase-mediated cleavage (Asp-61)
> ➤ Asparagine deamidation (Asn-52, Asn-66)

Loop Domain

BH4   **BH3**   **BH1**   **BH2**   **TM**   **Bcl-xL**

Fig. 5. Post-translational modification of Bcl-xL. There are three types of post-translational modifications of Bcl-xL, phosphorylation, cleavage, and asparagine deamidation targeted to the loop domain. *JNK*, Jun N-terminal kinase

Our observations indicate that Bcl-xL is deamidated in human liver tissues and, importantly, that Bcl-xL deamidation is significantly lower in HCC than in normal or adjacent nontumor liver tissues [18]. In general, asparagine deamidation results in the formation of isoaspartate, which can dramatically affect the conformation of the polypeptide and its biological function. Indeed, Devermann et al. [19] recently demonstrated that Bcl-xL deamidation caused a complete loss of Bcl-xL function. Therefore, our findings suggest that the suppression of Bcl-xL deamidation may be one of the mechanisms by which HCC acquires a survival advantage in vivo.

Conclusion

In conclusion, conditional deletion of the *bcl-x* gene revealed that Bcl-xL is an important apoptosis antagonist in hepatocytes. Transformed hepatocytes may acquire resistance to apoptosis and a survival advantage by suppressing the deamidation of Bcl-xL, as well as by increasing its expression.

References

1. Gross A, McDonnell JM, Korsmeyer SJ (1999) BCL-2 family members and the mitochondria in apoptosis. Genes Dev 13:1899–1911
2. Veis DJ, Sorenson CM, Shutter JR, Korsmeyer SJ (1993) Bcl-2 deficient mice demonstrate fulminant lymphoid apoptosis, polycystic kidneys, and hypopigmented hair. Cell 75:229–240
3. Print CG, Loveland KL, Gibson L, Meehan T, Stylianou A, Wreford N, De Kretser D, Metcalf D, Kontgen F, Adams JM, Cory S (1998) Apoptosis regulator Bcl-w is essential for spermatogenesis but appears otherwise redundant. Proc Natl Acad Sci USA 95: 12424–12431

4. Ross AJ, Waymire KG, Moss JE, Parlow AF, Skinner MK, Russell LD, MacGregor GR (1998) Testicular degeneration in Bclw-deficient mice. Nat Genet 18:251–256

5. Hamasaki A, Sendo F, Nakayama K, Ishida N, Negishi I, Nakayama K, Hatakeyama S (1998) Accelerated neutrophil apoptosis in mice lacking A1-a, a subtype of the bcl-2-related A1 gene. J Exp Med 188:1985–1992

6. Russell HR, Lee Y, Miller HL, Zhao J, McKinnon PJ (2002) Murine ovarian development is not affected by inactivation of the Bcl-2 family member Diva. Mol Cell Biol 22: 6866–6870

7. Motoyama N, Wang F, Roth KA, Sawa H, Nakayama K, Nakayama K, Negishi I, Senju S, Zhang Q, Fujii S, Loh DY (1995) Massive cell death of immature hematopoietic cells and neurons in Bcl-x-deficient mice. Science 267:1506–1510

8. Rinkenberger JL, Horning S, Klocke B, Roth K, Korsmeyer SJ (2000) Mcl-1 deficiency results in peri-implantation embryonic lethality. Genes Dev 14:23–27

9. Kren BT, Trembley JH, Krajewski S, Behrens TW, Reed JC, Steer CJ (1996) Modulation of apoptosis-associated genes bcl-2, bcl-x, and bax during rat liver regeneration. Cell Growth Differ 12:1633–1642

10. Tzung SP, Fausto N, Hockenbery DM (1997) Expression of Bcl-2 family during liver regeneration and identification of Bcl-x as a delayed early response gene. Am J Pathol 150:1985–1995

11. Hong F, Jaruga B, Kim WH, Radaeva S, El-Assal ON, Tian Z, Nguyen VA, Gao B (2002) Opposing roles of STAT1 and STAT3 in T cell-mediated hepatitis: regulation by SOCS. J Clin Invest 110:1503–1513

12. Kanegae Y, Lee G, Sato Y, Tanaka M, Nakai M, Sakaki T, Sugano S, Saito I (1995) Efficient gene activation in mammalian cells by using recombinant adenovirus expressing site-specific Cre recombinase. Nucleic Acids Res 23:3816–3821

13. Takehara T, Liu X, Fujimoto J, Friedman SL, Takahashi T (2001) Expression and role of Bcl-xL in human hepatocellular carcinomas. Hepatology 34:55–61

14. Poruchynsky MS, Wang EE, Rudin CM, Blagosklonny MV, Fojo T (1998) Bcl-xL is phosphorylated in malignant cells following microtubule disruption. Cancer Res 58: 3331–3338

15. Robinson AB, Rudd CJ (1974) Deamidation of glutaminyl and asparaginyl residues in peptides and proteins. Curr Top Cell Regul 8:247–295

16. Aswad DW, Paranandi MV, Schurter BT (2000) Isoaspartate in peptides and proteins: formation, significance, and analysis. J Pharm Biomed Anal 21:1129–1136

17. Robinson NE (2002) Protein deamidation. Proc Natl Acad Sci USA 99:5283–5288

18. Takehara T, Takahashi H (2000) Bcl-xL is posttranslationally deamidated at asparagine residues (abstract). FASEB J 15:A1517

19. Deverman BE, Cook BL, Manson SR, Niederhoff RA, Langer EM, Rosová I, Kulans LA, Fu X, Weinberg JS, Heinecke JW, Roth KA, Weintraub SJ (2002) Bcl-xL deamidation is a critical switch in the regulation of the response to DNA damage. Cell 111:51–62

Dedifferentiation and Proliferation of Hepatocellular Carcinoma: From Early to Advanced

MASAMICHI KOJIRO

Summary. It has been clarified that tumor proliferation is closely related to tumor cell dedifferentiation in hepatocellular carcinoma (HCC) at the early stage. Most small HCCs at the early stage consist solely of well-differentiated cancerous tissues and retain portal tracts inside. In the process of dedifferentiation, less-defferentiated HCC tissues generate in well-differentiated HCCs and they often show a "nodule-in-nodule" appearance, with a clear boundary, when less-differentiated HCC tissue is proliferating in an expansive fashion. Clinically, such a "nodule-in-nodule" appearance is easily appreciated by the examination of imagines. The areas of less-differentiated cancerous tissues inside the well-differentiated HCCs increase in size along with increases in tumor size, and, eventually, well-differentiated tumor nodules are completely replaced by less-differentiated cancerous tissues when the tumors reach around 3.0 cm in diameter. Thus, a "nodule-in-nodule" appearance is regarded as the morphologic marker of the multistep progression of tumor dedifferentiation in HCC, and various factors, such as p53, transforming growth factor (TGF)-α cyclooxygenase (COX)-2, vascular endothelial growth factor (VEGF), and others seem to be involved in the dedifferentiation process.

Key words. Hepatocellular carcinoma, Small HCC, Early HCC, Dedifferentiation, Nodule-in-nodule

Introduction

In addition to the remarkable advances that have been made in various diagnostic imaging techniques, the establishment of follow-up systems for populations at high risk of developing hepatocellular carcinoma (HCC) has enabled the diagnosis of HCC in the early stage. Based on extensive pathological studies of various-sized resected HCCs and biopsy materials from minute HCCs in the early stage, it has been clarified that the majority of small HCCs in the early stage are well differentiated [1–3]. Furthermore, studies of resected HCCs that show more than two different histologic grades have also clarified that when small well-differentiated HCCs increase in size, foci of less-differentiated cancerous tissues generate in them and increase in area until they totally replace the well-differentiated HCC tissues [4,5].

Department of Pathology, Kurume University School of Medicine, 67 Asahi-machi, Kurume 830-0011, Japan

Here, the evolution of HCC from early to advanced is described from the point of view of pathology.

Morphologic Characteristics of Early HCC

Grossly, small HCCs up to around 2 cm in diameter are classified as either distinctly nodular type or indistinctly nodular type. Many small HCCs of around 1.0–1.5 cm in diameter are indistinctly nodular and show a vaguely nodular appearance. They retain the basic architecture of the background cirrhotic liver in varying degrees and have an indistinct margin [6] (Fig. 1). Most of them are hypovascular on angiography. On the other hand, the distinctly nodular type shows a clear nodule, frequently with a fibrous capsule and fibrous septa, and is larger than the indistinctly nodular type. The average tumor size of indistinctly nodular HCCs is 11.9 ± 3.3 (SD) mm which is significantly smaller than the average size, 16.0 ± 3.3 (SD) mm, of the distinctly nodular type.

Histologically, about 70% of distinctly nodular HCCs are already moderately differentiated, despite the small tumor size. However, most indistinctly nodular HCCs are uniformly composed of well-differentiated cancerous tissues, and the well-differentiated cancer cells proliferate as if they are replacing the liver cell cords at the tumor-nontumor boundary, without forming a capsule. Well-differentiated HCCs are characterized by increased cell density, with an increased nuclear/cytoplasmic ratio, and increased cytoplasmic eosinophilia, compared with the surrounding non-cancerous tissue, and they have an irregular thin-trabecular pattern with a frequent

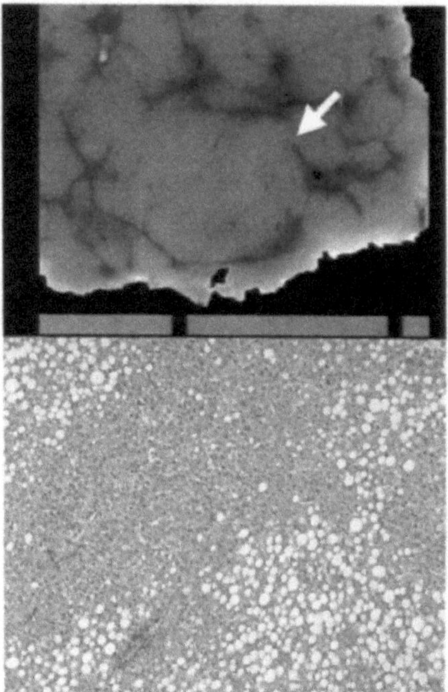

Fig. 1. Small hepatocellular carcinoma of indistinctly nodular type (early HCC). The tumor is vaguely nodular, with an indistinct margin (*arrow*) and consists of the uniform distribution of well-differentiated HCC tissue. In this case, there is marked diffuse fatty change in the cancer. (HE stain, ×50)

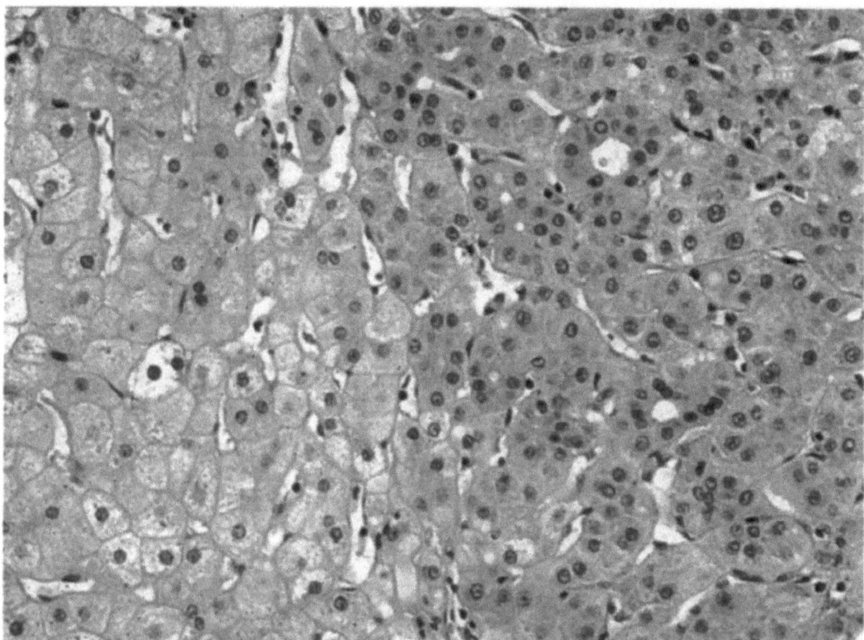

Fig. 2. Tumor-nontumor boundary of well-differentiated HCC of indistinctly nodular type (early HCC). Well-differentiated HCC (*right half of Fig.*) is characterized by increased cell density, an irregular trabecular pattern with occasional pseudoglandular pattern, and increased cytoplasmic staining, compared with the surrounding non-cancerous tissue. At the boundary, the cancer cells are proliferating in a replacing pattern as if they are replacing the surrounding liver cell cords, without forming a fibrous capsule. (HE stain, ×400)

pseudoglandular pattern (Fig. 2). Diffuse fatty change is observed in about 40% of them, and the frequency of this feature declines along with an increase of tumor size [7]. Tumor invasion into the portal vein branches and intrahepatic metastasis are rare in the indistinctly nodular type, but they are observed in 27% and 10%, respectively, of the distinctly nodular type. Thus, small HCCs of the indistinctly nodular type may be called "carcinoma in situ" of the liver, or its equivalent, and they are designated as "early HCC" in Japan. However, many of these "early HCCs" tend to be diagnosed as high-grade dysplastic nodules by Western pathologists. In the differentiation of early HCC from high-grade dysplastic nodules, the presence of stromal invasion, which is characterized by varying degrees of tumor cell invasion into the portal tracts inside the tumor, is very helpful [8] (Fig. 3).

Replacement of Well-Differentiated Cancerous Tissues by Less-Differentiated Cancerous Tissues in Early HCCs

In about 20% of small HCCs up to 2 cm in diameter, the tumor nodules consist of a mixture of different histologic grades, from well-differentiated to moderately differentiated, and the moderately differentiated cancerous tissues are located within the

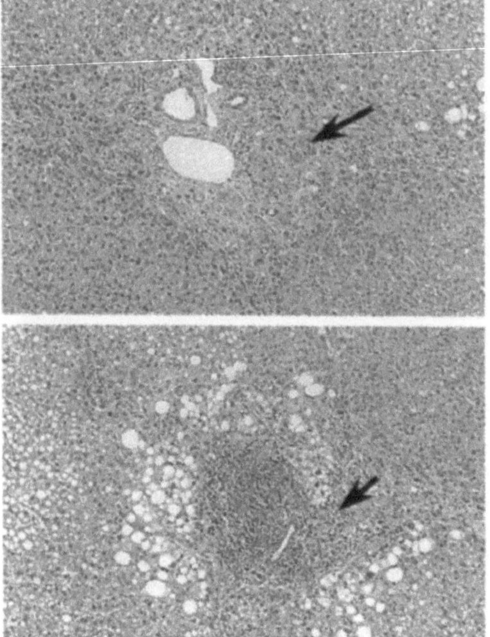

Fig. 3. Stromal invasion. Cancer cells are invading the portal tracts retained in early HCC (*arrows*). The presence of stromal invasion is often helpful for differentiating well-differentiated HCC from high-grade dysplastic nodules. (HE stain, ×80)

well-differentiated cancerous tissues. The areas of well-differentiated cancerous tissues diminish in size along with an increase of tumor size. Eventually, moderately and/or poorly differentiated cancerous tissues completely replace the well-differentiated cancerous tissues, and it is uncommon to find well-differentiated cancerous tissues in tumors larger than 3 cm.

"Nodule-in-Nodule" Appearance

When well-differentiated HCC nodules contain less-differentiated cancer tissue with a clear boundary, they often show a "nodule-in-nodule" appearance. In most small HCCs with a "nodule-in-nodule" appearance, the labeling index of proliferating-cell nuclear antigen (PCNA) is significantly higher in the less-differentiated inside nodule. This means that the proliferative activity of well-differentiated HCC is weaker than that of less-differentiated HCC. This has been proved by the study of well- and poorly differentiated HCC cell lines established from HCC with a "nodule-in-nodule" appearance [9]. In HCCs with a "nodule-in-nodule" appearance, overexpression of p53 protein is observed in the inner nodule, but not in the well-differentiated outer nodule in about 30% of the tumors [10]. On the other hand, overexpression of transforming growth factor (TGF)-α and cyclooxyenase (COX)-2 is observed in the outer nodule, but their expressions are weak in the less-differentiated inner nodule [11,12]. Thus, it is predicted that abnormalities of p53, TGF-alpha, COX-2, and other, unknown, factors may be involved in the differentiation process of well-differentiated HCC.

The most typical "nodule-in-nodule" appearance can be appreciated when well-differentiated HCCs with fatty change contain less-differentiated cancer tissues

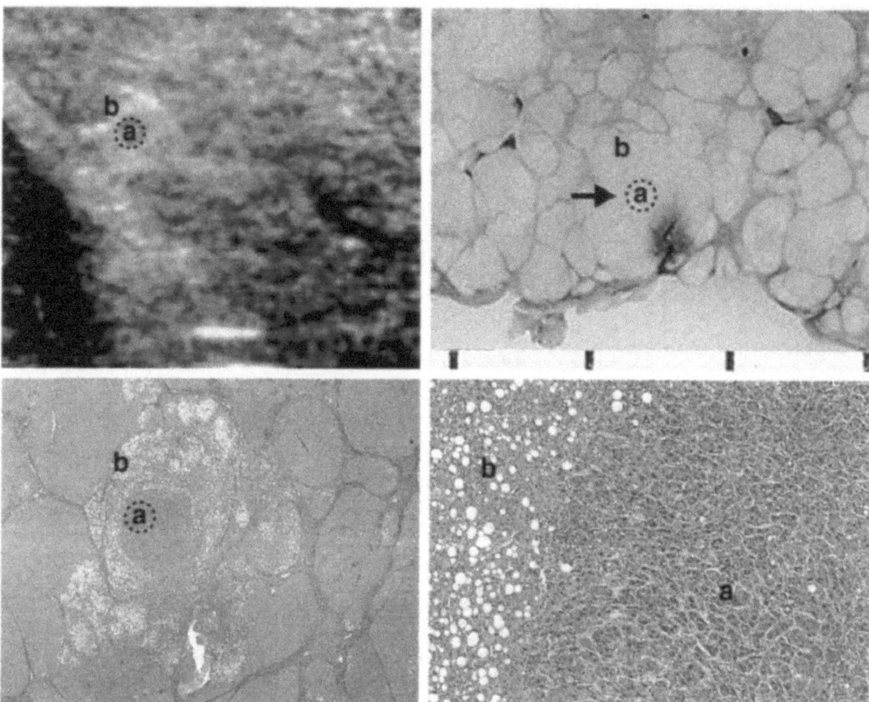

Fig. 4. Early HCC with "nodule-in-nodule" appearance. A small HCC was detected as a hyperechoic nodule, with a minute hypoechoic nodule inside, by ultrasonography. The tumor nodule, which has an indistinct margin, is 1.2 × 1.0 cm in size, and contains a minute nodule (*arrow*). The outer nodule consists of well-differentiated HCC with diffuse fatty change, and the inner nodule consists of moderately differentiated HCC with no fatty change. (HE stain, ×80)

without fatty change, and such tumors are detected as a hyperechoic nodule containing a well-demarcated hypoechoic nodule by ultrasonography (Fig. 4). According to follow-up observations, the hypoechoic nodule within the hyperechoic nodule gradually increases in size along with tumor growth, and eventually replaces the hyperechoic area. Such a transition in imaging findings reflects the progression of the dedifferentiation phenomenon in well-differentiated HCC, from early to advanced cancer. In cases of so-called "slow-growing hepatoma", which grows very slowly for months or even for years, serial biopsy studies have revealed that most of them stay in a well-differentiated condition until they start growing rapidly. Thus, it is assumed that the dediffrentiation caused by the replacement of well-differentiated cancer tissues by less-differentiated ones, which generate in well-differentiated cancer nodules, is closely related to tumor proliferation.

Monoclonal Dedifferentiation of Well-Differentiated HCC

The author's group has established a well-differentiated HCC cell line (HAK-1A) and a poorly differentiated HCC cell line (HAK-1B) from a resected small HCC showing a "nodule-in-nodule" appearance, with a clear boundary between the well-differentiated

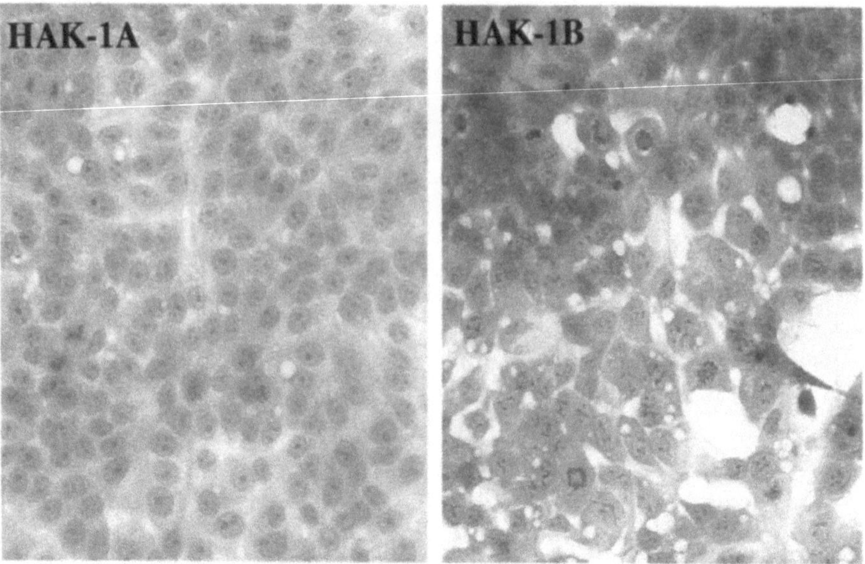

Fig. 5. Two distinct cell lines derived from HCC with a "nodule-in-nodule" appearance. Well-differentiated HAK-1A cells are derived from well-differentiated HCC tissue, and poorly differentiated HAK-1B cells are derived from poorly differentiated HCC inside the well-differentiated tumor. HAK-1B cells show rapid growth and their doubling time is only one-third of that of HAK-1A. (HE stain, ×400)

and poorly differentiated cancer tissues [9] (Fig. 5). These two cell lines show morphologically and biologically different characteristics: the doubling time of HAK-1A is approximately three times longer than that of HAK-1B; the DNA ploidy pattern is diploid in HAK-1A, but aneuploid in HAK-1B; and HAK-1B is easily transplantable to nude mice, while HAK-1A is not, because of its weak proliferative activity. Chromosome analysis revealed many different abnormalities in the two cell lines, in which, however, two identical structural abnormalities (2q+ and 17p+) were identified. In addition, nucleotide sequence analysis of exon 7 of the p53 gene showed an identical point mutation of p53 at codon 242 (Fig. 6). These findings strongly suggest that the two cell lines have the same clonal origin, and that the HAK-1B cells, which are poorly differentiated, might have developed from the dedifferentiation of the well-differentiated HAK-1A cells. Therefore, in an HCC nodule consisting of more than two histologic grades, it is conceivable that the less-differentiated cancer cells could be generated via the dedifferentiation of the well-differentiated cells, due to various mechanisms .

Evolution of Angioarchitecture in HCC from Early to Advanced

Although HCC is one of the typical hypervascular tumors, it is known that the majority of early HCCs are not depicted as hypervascular tumors by angiography and contrast imagings, whereas most small HCCs of the distinctly nodular type are detected as hypervascular tumors despite their small tumor size. Such different angiographic patterns in early HCC could be explained by the following three features. (1) Insuffi-

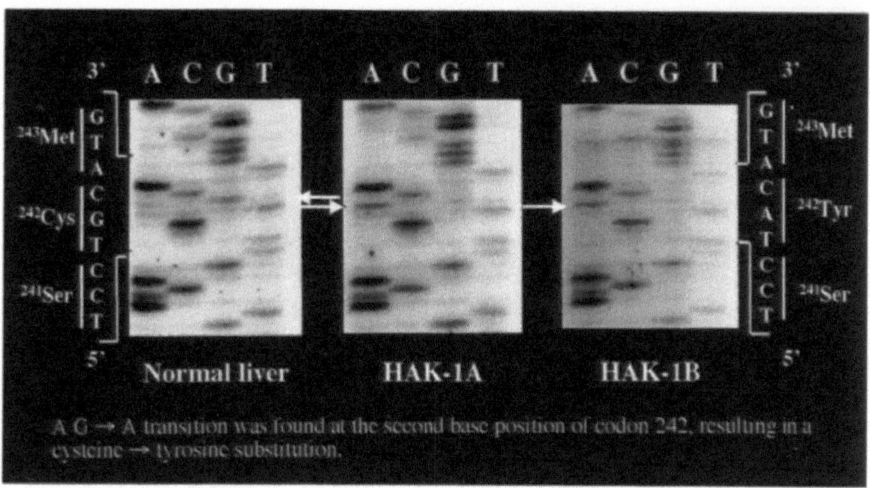

Fig. 6. Despite prominent morphologic and biologic differences between HAK-1A and HAK-1B cells, both cell lines have an identical point mutation of p53 at codon 242. They also have two identical chromosomal abnormalities. Accordingly, the two cell lines are considered to be monoclonal in origin, and it is suggested that HAK-1B cells seem to have been derived from HAK-1A

cient development of unpaired arteries [13]; the number of unpaired arteries (arterial tumor vessels) per square millimeter in tumors that are less than 1.5 cm in size is significantly lower than that in advanced HCCs, but the number becomes the same as that in advanced tumors when the tumor reaches about 2 cm in diameter. (2) Lack of a fibrous capsule (replacing growth at the tumor-nontumor boundaries). (3) Incomplete vascularization of sinusoid-like blood spaces. In moderately differentiated HCCs, the endothelial cells of the blood spaces are immunohistochemically positive for CD34, and a laminin-positive reaction, corresponding to a basement membrane-like structure, is also observed along the blood spaces (Fig. 7). In many early HCCs, however, positive reaction to CD34 is weak [9,14–19]. Thus, it can be said that vascularization of the blood spaces is still incomplete in early HCCs. In tumors with a "nodule-in-nodule" appearance, inner nodules consisting of moderately differentiated tumor are frequently depicted as hypervascular nodules within a hypovascular tumor. In fact, unpaired arteries and sinusoidal capillarization are well developed in the moderately differentiated HCC in the inner nodule compared with the development in the surrounding well-differentiated cancerous tissues.

Conclusions

The pathological evolution of HCC from an early to an advanced form progresses in a multistep fashion, along with molecular events. According to the findings that small HCCs in the early stage are mostly well-differentiated and have weak proliferative activity, with infrequent portal vein invasion and intrahepatic metastasis, it is important to detect and treat HCCs in the early stage to expect better prognosis, although recurrence due to multicentric occurrence cannot be prevented.

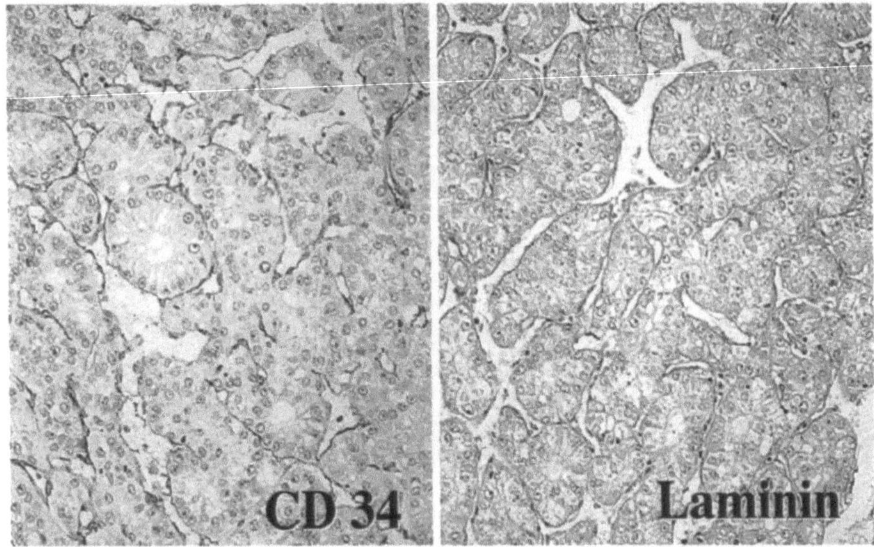

Fig. 7. Sinusoidal capillarization in moderately differentiated HCC. Sinusoidal endothelial cells are immunohistochemically positive for CD34 and laminin. (Immunostain, ×200)

References

1. Kanai T, Hirohashi S, Upton M, Noguchi M, Kishi K, Makuuchi M, Yamasaki S, Hasegawa H, Takayasu K, Moriyama N, Shimosato Y (1987) Pathology of small hepatocellular carcinoma. A proposal for a new gross classification. Cancer 60:810–819
2. Kondo Y, Niwa Y, Akikusa B, Takazawa H, Okabayashi A (1983) A histopathologic study of early hepatocellular carcinoma. Cancer 52:687–692
3. Kojiro M, Nakashima O (1999) Histopathologic evaluation of hepatocellular carcinoma with special reference to small early stage tumor. Semin Liver Dis 19:287–296
4. Kenmochi K, Sugihara S, Kojiro M (1987) Relationship of histologic grade of hepatocellular carcinoma (HCC) to tumor size, and demonstration of tumor cells of multiple different grades in a single small HCC. Liver 7:18–26.
5. Sugihara S, Nakashima O, Kojiro M, Majima Y, Tanaka M, Tanikawa K (1992) The morphologic transition in hepatocellular carcinoma. A comparison of the individual histological features disclosed by ultrasound-guided fine-needle biopsy with those of autopsy. Cancer 70:1488–1492
6. Nakashima O, Sugihara S, Kage M, Kojiro M (1995) Pathomorphologic characteristics of small hepatocellular carcinoma: a special reference to small hepatocellular carcinoma with indistinct margins. Hepatology 22:101–105
7. Kutami R, Nakashima Y, Nakashima O, Shiota K, Kojiro M (2000) Pathomorphologic study on the mechanism of fatty change in small hepatocellular carcinoma of humans. J Hepatol 33:282–289
8. Tomizawa M, Kondo F, Kondo Y (1995) Growth patterns and interstitial invasion of small hepatocellular carcinoma. Pathol Int 45:352–358
9. Yano H, Iemura A, Fukuda K, Mizoguchi A, Haramaki M, Kojiro M (1993) Establishment of two distinct human hepatocellular carcinoma cell lines from a single nodule showing clonal dedifferentiation of cancer cells. Hepatology 18: 320–327

10. Nakashima Y, Hsia C, Yuwen H, Ninemura M, Nakashima O, Kojiro M, Tabor E (1998) P53 overexpression in small hepatocellular carcinoma containing two different histologic grades. Int J Oncol 12:455–459

11. Morimitsu Y, Hsia C, Kojiro M, Tabor E (1995) Nodules of less-differentiated tumor within or adjacent to hepatocellular carcinoma. Relative expression of transforming growth factor-α and its receptor in the different areas of tumor. Hum Pathol 26:1126–1132

12. Koga H, Sakisaka S, Ohishi M, Kawaguchi T, Taniguchi E, Sasatomi K, Hara M, Kusaba T, Tanaka M, Kimura R, Nakashima Y, Nakashima O, Kojiro M, Kurohiji T, Sata M (1999) Expression of cyclooxygenase-2 in human hepatocellular carcinoma: relevance to tumor dedifferentiation. Hepatology 29:688–696

13. Nakashima Y, Nakashima O, Hsia C, Tabor E (1999) Vascularization of small hepatocellular carcinomas: correlation with differentiation. Liver 19:12–18

14. Park Y, Yang C, Cubukcu O, Thung S, Theise N (1998) Neoangiogenesis and sinusoidal "capillarization" in dysplastic nodules of the liver. Am J Surg Pathol 22:271–274

15. Kimura H, Nakajima T, Kagawa K, Deguchi T, Kakusui M, Katagishi T, Okanoue T, Kashima K, Ashihara T (1998) Angiogenesis in hepatocellular carcinoma as evaluated by CD34 immunohistochemistry. Liver 18:14–19

16. Maeda T, Adachi E, Kajiyama K, Takenaka K, Honda H, Sugimachi K, Tsuneyoshi M (1995) CD34 expression in endothelial cells of small hepatocellular carcinoma: its correlation with tumor progression and angiographic findings. J Gastroenterol Hepatol 10:650–654

17. Enzan H, Himeno H, Iwamura S, Onishi S, Saibara T, Yamamoto Y, Hara H (1994) α-Smooth muscle actin-positive perisinusoidal stromal cells in human hepatocellular carcinoma. Hepatology 19:895–903

18. Sakamoto M, Ino Y, Fuji T, Hirohashi S (1993) Phenotype changes in tumor vessels associated with the progression of hepatocellular carcinoma. Jpn J Clin Oncol 23:98–104

19. Kin M, Torimura T, Ueno T, Inuzuka S, Tanikawa K (1994) Sinusoidal capillarization in small hepatocellular carcinoma. Pathol Int 44:771–778

Genome-Wide Analysis of Gene Expression in Hepatocellular Carcinoma

Taro Yamashita, Shuichi Kaneko, Masao Honda, and Kenichi Kobayashi

Summary. Hepatocellular carcinoma (HCC) is one of the most common malignant tumors worldwide. The major risk factor associated with HCC is chronic hepatitis resulting from infection with hepatitis B virus (HBV) or hepatitis C virus (HCV), but the molecular mechanisms of hepatocarcinogenesis still remain obscure. To elucidate the mechanisms of hepatocarcinogenesis, serial analysis of gene expression (SAGE) was performed in HBV-related HCC tissues (HCC-B), HCV-related HCC tissues (HCC-C), and associated noncancerous tissues. A total of 157,849 transcripts were generated, including 35,360 unique tags. Transcripts upregulated in the HCC-B library were those encoding HBV X protein, ESTs, osteonectin, and many unknown proteins. Transcripts upregulated in the HCC-C library were those encoding interferon gamma inducible proteins, oxidative stress-inducible proteins, glypican 3, and diubiquitin. Downregulation of genes associated with drug detoxification was observed in both HCC-B and HCC-C tissues. To evaluate the differential gene expression changes identified by SAGE in other HCCs, we prepared glass slides containing the sets of genes detected by SAGE, and performed cDNA microarray analysis on HCC-B and HCC-C tissues. Hierarchical clustering of these cDNA microarray data clearly distinguished HCC-B tissues from HCC-C tissues, validating the SAGE data. Thus, the combination of SAGE and cDNA microarray with human genome databases clarified differential gene expression patterns between HCC-B and HCC-C, and provided novel candidate genes to decipher the molecular mechanisms of carcinogenesis in chronic viral hepatitis.

Key words. Gene expression profile, Hepatitis virus, Hepatocellular carcinoma, Serial analysis of gene expression, cDNA microarray

Introduction

Hepatocellular carcinoma (HCC) is one of the most common malignancies in the world. The major risk factor associated with hepatocarcinogenesis is chronic hepatitis (CH) resulting from infection with hepatitis B virus (HBV) or hepatitis C virus (HCV) [1]. Molecular approaches have shown that several oncogenes and tumor sup-

Department of Gastroenterology, Kanazawa University Graduate School of Medicine, 13-1 Takara-Machi, Kanazawa 920-8641, Japan

pressor genes, and their mutations, are associated with hepatocarcinogenesis, including *p53* mutations [2–5], *p16* alterations [6], and so on. However, these studies have focused on only a limited number of genes associated with carcinogenesis in other types of cancers, and have not revealed the biological nature of HCC precisely.

Serial analysis of gene expression (SAGE) is a nonbiased method used to monitor gene expression changes, including unknown genes, and potentially describes all genes expressed in tissue [7,8]. To gain insight into the molecular mechanisms of hepatocarcinogenesis, we performed SAGE in a chronic hepatitis B (CH-B) tissue and an HBV-related HCC (HCC-B) tissue from a patient, and compared these with the reported SAGE libraries of a normal liver (NL) tissue, a CH-C tissue, and an HCC-C tissue [9,10].

Patients, Materials, and Methods

Samples

Two normal human liver tissue samples were derived from surgically resected tissues of colon-cancer metastasis, and the samples were obtained from the portion unaffected by the cancer. All HCC tissues and corresponding noncancerous liver tissues were derived from ten patients who had undergone surgical resection of the tumor for treatment of a solitary HCC. Five HCC-B samples were obtained from patients with positive serum hepatitis B surface antigen, determined using a commercial enzyme immunoassay (Dainabot, Tokyo, Japan). Five HCC-C samples were obtained from patients with positive serum HCV-RNA, determined using Amplicor monitor analysis (Roche Diagnostic System, Branchburg, NZ). All procedures and risks were explained verbally to the patients, as well as being explained in a written consent form.

SAGE

Total RNA was extracted from the homogenized sample, using a ToTally RNA extraction kit (Ambion, Austin, TX, USA). Polyadenylated RNA was extracted using a MicroPoly (A) Pure kit (Ambion) according to the manufacturer's protocol. A total of 2.5 μg of mRNA was used for SAGE. The SAGE protocol was as described previously [7,11]. SAGE libraries were sequenced at random, using ABI PRISM 373 and 377 DNA sequencers and a BigDye Terminator Cycle Sequencing Kit (PE Biosystems, Foster City, CA, USA). All sequence files were analyzed with the SAGE 2000 software kindly gifted by Drs. Kenneth W. Kinzler and Bert Vogelstein. The gene expression profiles of the CH-B and HCC-B tissues were compared with those of an NL tissue, a CH-C tissue, and an HCC tissue we described previously [9,10]. The statistical significance of differences between samples was calculated using the Monte-Carlo simulation. Annotation of each tag was performed by the use of a SAGE tag to the gene mapping web site (http://www.ncbi.nlm.nih.gov/SAGE/index.cgi).

cDNA Microarray

From genes that were up- or downregulated more than fivefold in the HCC-B or HCC-C libraries compared with the NL library, 20 genes were selected at random, and added to the 1080 genes (Kanazawa Liver Chip Ver. 3). Corresponding cDNA clones were obtained by reverse transcription-polymerase chain reaction (RT-PCR) amplification using gene-specific primers and a TOPO TA cloning kit (Invitrogen, Carlsbad, CA, USA) according to the manufacturer's instructions. All clones were sequence-verified using the ABI PRISM 373 and 377 DNA sequencer and BigDye Terminator Cycle Sequencing Kit (PE Biosystems). PCR products amplified from clones were spotted on glass slides using SPBIO 2000 (Hitachi Software, Fukuoka, Japan). To normalize varying efficiencies of labeling and detection, control genes (encoding Renilla and Firefly luciferase) were spotted in each slide. Extracted total RNAs were amplified by antisense RNA amplification, and 5 μg of amplified RNA was used for fluorescence labeling by Cy3 or Cy5 (detailed protocols have been described previously [12]). The labeled probes were purified on Microcon 30 columns (Millipore, Bedford, MA, USA), and hybridization was performed as previously described [13]. The same amplified RNA obtained from a normal liver tissue was used as reference in all hybridizations. Quantitative assessment of the signals was carried out using ScanArray 3000 (General Scanning, Watertown, MA, USA), followed by image analysis using QuantArray software (General Scanning) as per the manufacturer's protocol. The obtained data were log-transferred, normalized, mean-centered, and applied to average linkage clustering. Cluster analysis was performed using TreeView software (http://rana.Stanford.EDU/software/).

Results

SAGE Profiles

In addition to the 94,580 tags of three SAGE libraries we reported previously (derived from an NL tissue, a CH-C tissue, and an HCC-C tissue), 30,543 tags were obtained from the CH-B library and 32,726 tags from the HCC-B library, and a total of 157,849 tags were analyzed. These 157,849 tags included 35,360 unique tags, and at least 1250 tags did not match any of the nonredundant transcripts reported in GenBank thus far (data not shown). Scatter plots of the distribution of all tags in each library revealed that the gene expression patterns observed in the CH-B tissue were similar to those in the NL ($R^2 = 0.7585$) and CH-C tissues ($R^2 = 0.759$); however, they were most similar to the HCC-B tissue which originated from the CH-B tissue (Fig. 1). The plots were relatively scattered between the HCC-B and the NL tissues ($R^2 = 0.6634$), and between the HCC-B and the HCC-C tissues ($R^2 = 0.5829$). These data suggested the existence of distinct gene expression patterns in the CH-B tissue and the HCC-B tissue, caused by HBV infection.

Genes that were Differentially Expressed

Forty-nine genes were induced more than tenfold in the HCC-B tissue compared with the NL tissue. All of the transcripts induced more than tenfold are shown in Table 1. One of these did not exist in the reported human genome sequences and completely matched the sequence of the HBV genome corresponding to the *HBV-X* gene. Well-known transcripts upregulated in the HCC-B tissue were those encoding DEAD/H box

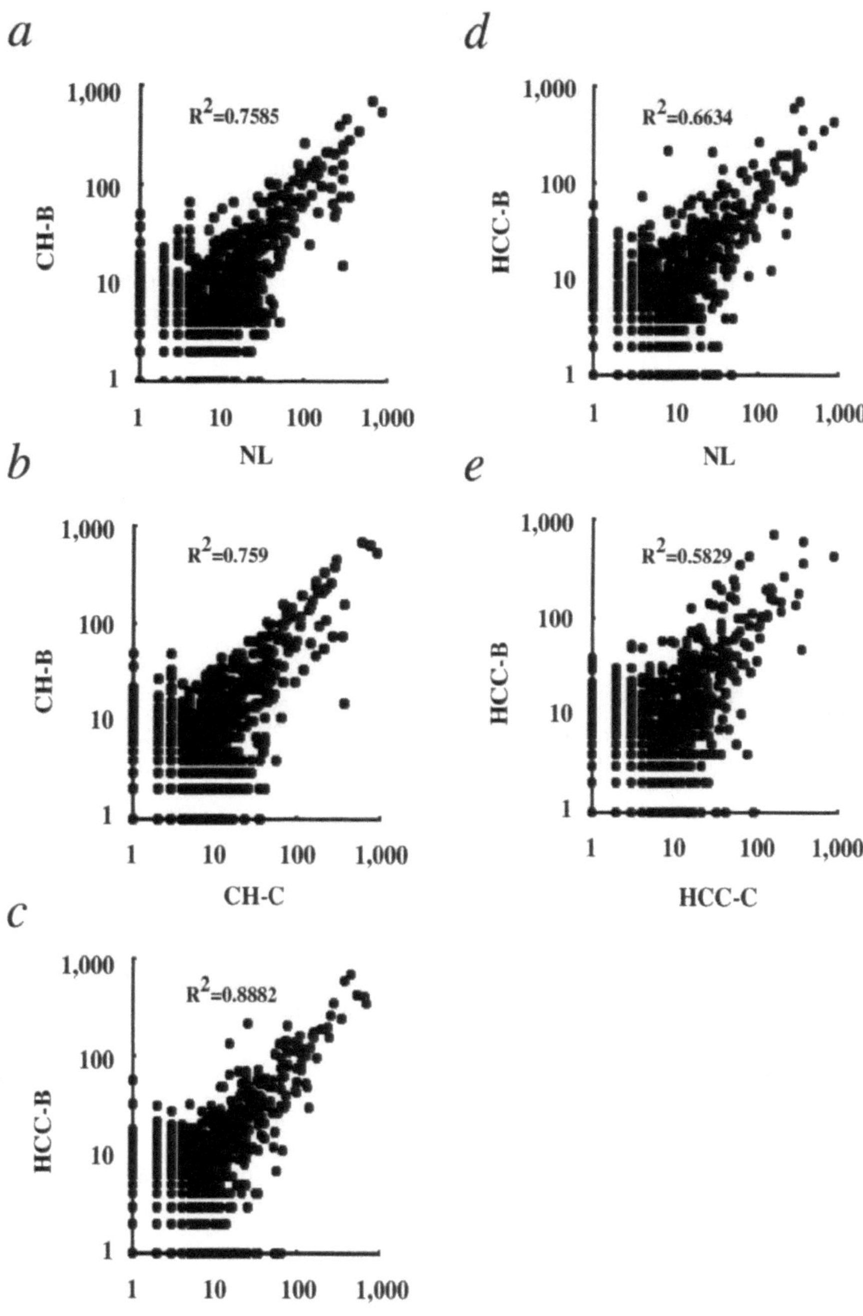

Fig. 1a–e. Distribution of tags in each serial analysis of gene expression (SAGE) library. The distribution of all SAGE tags in each library was plotted on a logarithmic scale. **a–c** The gene expression patterns in the chronic hepatitis B (*CH-B*) tissue were similar to those in the normal liver (*NL*; $R^2 = 0.7585$) and the chronic hepatitis C (*CH-C*; $R^2 = 0.759$), but were most similar to the hepatitis B virus-related hepatocellular carcinoma (*HCC-B*) tissues ($R^2 = 0.8882$). **d,e** The gene expression patterns in the HCC-B tissue were slightly different from those in the NL ($R^2 = 0.6634$) and the hepatitis C virus-related HCC (*HCC-C*) tissues ($R^2 = 0.5829$). These data suggested the existence of distinct gene expression patterns caused by hepatitis B virus (HBV) infection

Table 1. Genes induced in the HCC-B library compared with the NL library by SAGE

Fold	NL	CH-C	CH-B	HCC-C	HCC-B	Gene (GenBank accession number)
			Count			
58	0	1	1	7	58	No reliable match
39	0	0	37	0	39	No reliable match
33	0	0	1	0	33	Hepatitis B virus X protein (AY040627)
27	1	3	50	2	27	No reliable match
26.8	8	46	26	32	214	No reliable match
24	1	10	11	15	24	DEAD/H box polypeptide 5 (NM_004396)
21	0	2	9	0	21	EST similar to alpha-1-antitrypsin (T46850)
21	1	4	2	5	21	No reliable match
19	1	1	14	0	19	No reliable match
18	0	1	3	0	18	No reliable match
18	0	6	6	8	18	No reliable match
17.8	4	3	20	16	71	No reliable match
17	0	0	0	0	17	No reliable match
16	0	0	3	2	16	Glutathione peroxidase 2 (BE735523)
16	1	5	8	4	16	Multiple match
16	1	1	10	0	16	No reliable match
15.5	2	3	2	7	31	Multiple match
15	0	0	0	0	15	EST (T91234)
15	0	3	5	6	15	Ostenectin (BE677127)
15	1	0	9	0	15	No reliable match
14.5	2	18	19	1	29	No reliable match
14	0	2	2	1	14	EST (AF084559)
14	1	0	3	1	14	EST (AV662152)
14	1	3	6	3	14	Multiple match
13	0	0	1	4	13	EST (T51930)
13	0	1	0	0	13	Multiple match
13	0	1	7	2	13	Microsomal triglyceride transfer protein (BF511063)
12	0	0	1	1	12	EST (T24502)
12	0	1	1	2	12	Multiple match
12	0	6	4	6	12	Defender against cell death 1 (BE881064)
12	1	0	1	4	12	EST (AV723833)
12	1	1	5	3	12	Multiple match
11	2	4	2	3	22	Multiple match
11	2	0	14	3	22	Multiple match
11	0	0	1	6	11	Multiple match
11	0	2	2	1	11	EST (W72996)
11	0	2	5	0	11	Ribosomal protein S27-like (AW139036)
11	0	3	5	3	11	Cyclin D1 (N72201)
11	1	2	1	4	11	Multiple match
11	1	2	0	2	11	Multiple match
11	1	1	2	0	11	EST similar to alpha-1-antitrypsin (T39894)
11	1	3	3	8	11	Multiple match
11	1	3	6	1	11	No reliable match
10	0	0	0	0	10	Multiple match
10	0	2	2	3	10	EST (T61571)
10	0	5	2	10	10	Multiple match
10	1	0	1	10	10	Multiple match
10	1	4	11	5	10	Multiple match
10	1	4	15	3	10	No reliable match

SAGE, serial analysis of gene expression; NL, normal liver; CH-C, chronic hepatitis C; CH-B, chronic hepatitis B; HCC-C, hepatitis C virus-related hepatocellular carcinoma; HCC-B, hepatitis B virus-related hepatocellualr carcinoma

polypeptide 5, osteonectin, and cyclin D1. Thirty-five genes were repressed more than tenfold in the HCC-B tissue compared with the NL tissue. All of the transcripts repressed more than tenfold are listed in Table 2. Two of these transcripts have not been deposited in GenBank thus far, but these two tags completely matched the reported human genome sequences, suggesting that all these downregulated transcripts were derived from the normal human genome. Most of the downregulated transcripts were those associated with drug detoxification, such as cytochrome P450 (CYP) IIIA4, -IVA11, and -IA2, and those associated with carbohydrate metabolism, such as aldolase B.

Combination of SAGE with cDNA Microarray

To evaluate the gene expression patterns identified by SAGE in other HCC tissues, four HCC-B tissues and four HCC-C tissues were homogenized, and total RNAs were extracted and used for cDNA microarray analysis. To clarify the relationship between each HCC tissue and the gene expression profile, we performed hierarchical clustering (Fig. 2). The resulting dendrogram showed two cluster branches—one comprising the HCC-B branch and the other the HCC-C branch—and clearly demonstrated an association of gene expression patterns with the virological features of HCC. Several genes were preferentially upregulated in HCC-B lesions compared with HCC-C lesions, such as those encoding tumor necrosis factor (TNF)-alpha, consistent with the SAGE data. However, the HBV genome, the most specific gene for HCC-B by SAGE analysis, was not always upregulated in HCC-B tissues. These data revealed the existence of a large variety of characteristics in HCC lesions, but cDNA microarray analysis could successfully distinguish HCC-B lesions from HCC-C lesions, revealing the usefulness of gene expression profiling in HCC classification.

Discussion

Many upregulated tags in HCC-B did not match the known or hypothetical genes annotated thus far. The reason why so many unknown tags were upregulated in the HCC-B library is unclear. Because most of the differentially expressed genes in the HCC-C library identified by SAGE were known genes [10], one hypothesis that could be postulated would be that HBV infection and its genome insertion might cause these strange gene expression changes. A recent study using HBV-Alu-PCR demonstrated that the HBV DNA sometimes integrated into cellular genes that were key regulators of cell proliferation and viability [14]. Another study demonstrated that chromosome instability was more prominent in HCC-B tissues than in HCC-C tissues [15]. The unknown tags detected here might also encode important unknown genes required for malignant transformation caused by HBV infection.

We found one tag upregulated in an HCC-B lesion that did not match any known human genes, and the sequence completely matched the *HBV X* gene. Previous reports have suggested that *HBV X* gene products with aberrant transactivation properties may play an important role in malignant transformation [16,17]. The upregulation of *HBV X* in the HCC-B lesion was consistent with previous reports [18,19], and strongly suggested the importance of *HBV X* in HBV-related hepatocarcinogenesis. Well-

Table 2. Genes repressed in the HCC-B library compared with the NL library by SAGE

Fold	NL	CH-C	CH-B	HCC-C	HCC-B	Gene (GenBank accession number)
			Count			
50	50	42	55	0	1	Cytochrome P450 IIIA4 (M13785)
34	34	10	14	7	1	Betaine-homocysteine methyltransferase (AY040627)
30	30	17	11	3	0	Cytochrome P450 IVA 11 (NM_000778)
25	25	25	14	0	0	Hepcidin antimicrobial peptide (AF309489)
23	23	5	1	12	0	MHC class I, C (AJ010748)
23	23	36	2	16	1	Multiple match
17	17	8	12	0	0	Solute carrier family 22 member 1 (X98332)
17	17	6	6	3	1	Multiple match
17	34	8	4	19	2	No reliable match
16	16	3	5	1	0	Glycine N-methyltransferase (NM_018960)
15	15	7	0	1	0	EST (AW296644)
14.5	29	36	1	19	2	No reliable match
13	13	4	2	0	0	IGFBP, acid labile subunit (NM_004970)
13	13	5	4	1	1	Multiple match
13	13	13	7	5	1	Acetyl-coenzyme A acetyltransferase 2 (NM_006111)
13	13	35	32	89	1	Multiple match
13	52	58	4	36	4	EST (BG00487)
12.1	145	80	52	14	12	Aldolase B, fructose-bisphosphate (H57841)
12	12	17	18	2	0	Cytochrome P450 IA 2 (T51930)
12	12	7	2	1	1	Dual specificity phosphatase 1 (BE675054)
12	12	5	3	21	1	Translation elongation factor 1 alpha 1 (R57843)
12	12	13	3	2	1	Multiple match
11	11	3	2	4	0	Glucose-6-phosphatase, transport protein 1 (BE779193)
11	11	10	3	0	0	EST (AW827199)
11	11	13	0	8	1	EST (BM469146)
10.5	42	31	31	29	4	Multiple match
10	10	4	0	1	0	Multiple match
10	10	6	4	1	0	Multiple match
10	10	15	8	0	0	Ficolin 3 (AV708328)
10	10	9	16	0	0	EST similar to cytochrome P450 IIIA (AV685278)
10	10	0	1	0	1	Multiple match
10	10	7	2	0	1	EST (BF194872)
10	10	7	3	15	1	EST (BM546595)
10	10	16	15	0	1	Multiple match
10	20	12	11	12	2	Alcohol dehydrogenase 4 pi polypeptide (R83422)

NL, normal liver; CH-C, chronic hepatitis C; CH-B, chronic hepatitis B; HCC-C, hepatitis C virus-related hepatocellular carcinoma; HCC-B, hepatitis B virus-related hepatocellular carcinoma; IGFBP, insulin like growth factor binding protein

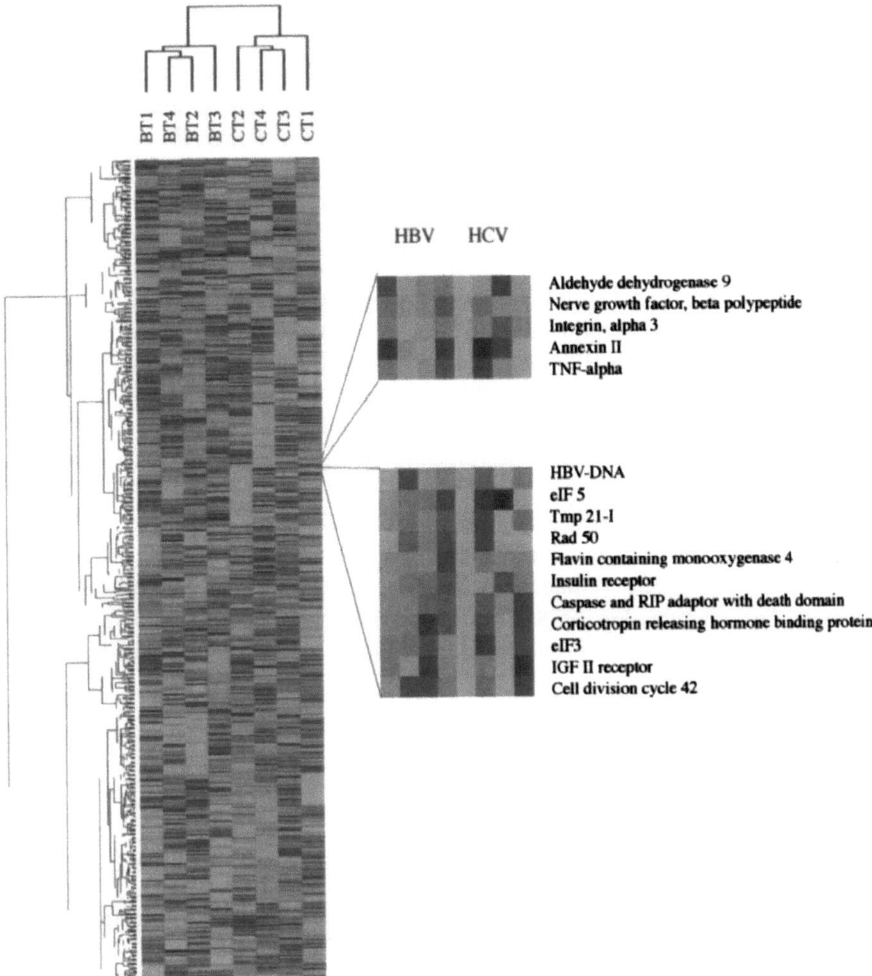

Fig. 2. cDNA microarray analysis. Hierarchical clustering of the gene expressions in eight HCC tissues (four HCC-B and four HCC-C) is shown. The *rows* represent individual genes, and the *columns* represent individual tissues, and the *color in each cell* reflects the expression levels of genes in the corresponding tissue. The resulting *dendrogram* shows two branches, one exactly corresponding to the HCC-B branch and one, to the HCC-C branch. Although heterogeneity of gene expressions existed in each tissue, genes encoding tumor necrosis factor (*TNF*)-alpha and hepatitis B virus (*HBV*) DNA were preferentially upregulated in HCC-B lesions. *eIF*, elongation initiation factor

known genes upregulated in the HCC-B tissue were those associated with cell-cycle regulation, transcription and translation, and protein degradation, such as cyclin D1, DEAD/H box polypeptide 5, and some proteasome subunits. Cyclin D1 is known as an oncogene, and is reported to be upregulated in HCC tissues [20], and to cause hepatocarcinogenesis in transgenic mice [21]. The upregulation of proteasome gene expression might cause proteolysis, which drives the cell cycle by degrading CDK inhibitors [22,23]. Thus, the gene expression changes identified here are consistent with the previous reports.

In this study, we selected genes that were differentially expressed in cancerous and noncancerous tissues by SAGE, and performed cDNA microarray analysis. By combining cDNA microarray analysis with SAGE, we could overcome the uncertainty of the SAGE tags and versatile patterns of expression in each HCC sample, and we identified the preferential upregulation of several genes in HCC-B lesions, including that of TNF-alpha. TNF-alpha is known as a pro-apoptotic cytokine, and is upregulated in hepatocytes by HBV X protein expression [24]. We previously reported the upregulation of pro-apoptotic genes in CH-B lesions compared with CH-C lesions [12], and it is possible that the cells comprising HCC-B tissue might overcome the pro-apoptotic effect of HBV infection or HBV genome integration. Thus, although a common feature of gene expression patterns in HCC-B lesions was difficult to detect by SAGE analysis alone, we could successfully distinguish HCC-B lesions from HCC-C lesions by applying cDNA microarray analysis, revealing the usefulness of microarray analysis in cancer classification.

In conclusion, we performed genome-wide analysis of gene expression in HCC-B lesions, clarified gene expression patterns specific for HCC-B lesions, and revealed novel genes that were differentially expressed in cancerous and noncancerous tissues. The combination of SAGE, cDNA microarray analysis, and the human genome database is a very powerful method to decipher the mechanisms of hepatocarcinogenesis.

References

1. Ozturk M (1999) Genetic aspects of hepatocellular carcinogenesis. Semin Liver Dis 19: 235–242
2. Oda T, Tsuda H, Scarpa A, Sakamoto M, Hirohashi S (1992) *p53* gene mutation spectrum in hepatocellular carcinoma. Cancer Res 52:6358–6364
3. Scorsone KA, Zhou YZ, Butel JS, Slagle BL (1992) p53 mutations cluster at codon 249 in hepatitis B virus-positive hepatocellular carcinomas from China. Cancer Res 52: 1635–1638
4. Hayashi H, Sugio K, Matsumata T, Adachi E, Takenaka K, Sugimachi K (1995) The clinical significance of p53 gene mutation in hepatocellular carcinomas from Japan. Hepatology 22:1702–1707
5. Minouchi K, Kaneko S, Kobayashi K (2002) Mutation of p53 gene in regenerative nodules in cirrhotic liver. J Hepatol 37:231–239
6. Tannapfel A, Busse C, Weinans L, Benicke M, Katalinic A, Geissler F, Hauss J, Wittekind C (2001) INK4a-ARF alterations and p53 mutations in hepatocellular carcinomas. Oncogene 20:7104–7109
7. Velculescu VE, Zhang L, Vogelstein B, Kinzler KW (1995) Serial analysis of gene expression. Science 270:484–487
8. Velculescu VE, Zhang L, Zhou W, Vogelstein J, Basrai MA, Bassett DE, Jr, Hieter P, Vogelstein B, Kinzler KW (1997) Characterization of the yeast transcriptome. Cell 88: 243–251
9. Yamashita T, Hashimoto S, Kaneko S, Nagai S, Toyoda N, Suzuki T, Kobayashi K, Matsushima K (2000) Comprehensive gene expression profile of a normal human liver. Biochem Biophys Res Commun 269:110–116

10. Yamashita T, Kaneko S, Hashimoto S, Sato T, Nagai S, Toyoda N, Suzuki T, Kobayashi K, Matsushima K (2001) Serial analysis of gene expression in chronic hepatitis C and hepatocellular carcinoma. Biochem Biophys Res Commun 282:647–654

11. Hashimoto S, Suzuki T, Dong HY, Yamazaki N, Matsushima K (1999) Serial analysis of gene expression in human monocytes and macrophages. Blood 94:837–844

12. Honda M, Kaneko S, Kawai H, Shirota Y, Kobayashi K (2001) Differential gene expression between chronic hepatitis B and C hepatic lesion. Gastroenterology 120:955–966

13. Kawai HF, Kaneko S, Honda M, Shirota Y, Kobayashi K (2001) Alpha-fetoprotein-producing hepatoma cell lines share common expression profiles of genes in various categories demonstrated by cDNA microarray analysis. Hepatology 33:676–691

14. Gozuacik D, Murakami Y, Saigo K, Chami M, Mugnier C, Lagorce D, Okanoue T, Urashima T, Brechot C, Paterlini–Brechot P (2001) Identification of human cancer-related genes by naturally occurring hepatitis B virus DNA tagging. Oncogene 20:6233–6240

15. Laurent-Puig P, Legoix P, Bluteau O, Belghiti J, Franco D, Binot F, Monges G, Thomas G, Bioulac-Sage P, Zucman-Rossi J (2001) Genetic alterations associated with hepatocellular carcinomas define distinct pathways of hepatocarcinogenesis. Gastroenterology 120:1763–1773

16. Cromlish JA (1996) Hepatitis B virus-induced hepatocellular carcinoma: possible roles for HBx. Trends Microbiol 4:270–274

17. Murakami S (1999) Hepatitis B virus X protein: structure, function and biology. Intervirology 42:81–99

18. Su Q, Schroder CH, Hofmann WJ, Otto G, Pichlmayr R, Bannasch P (1998) Expression of hepatitis B virus X protein in HBV-infected human livers and hepatocellular carcinomas. Hepatology 27:1109–1120

19. Chen WN, Oon CJ, Leong AL, Koh S, Teng SW (2000) Expression of integrated hepatitis B virus X variants in human hepatocellular carcinomas and its significance. Biochem Biophys Res Commun 276:885–892

20. Joo M, Kang YK, Kim MR, Lee HK, Jang JJ (2001) Cyclin D1 overexpression in hepatocellular carcinoma. Liver 21:89–95

21. Deane NG, Parker MA, Aramandla R, Diehl L, Lee WJ, Washington MK, Nanney LB, Shyr Y, Beauchamp RD (2001) Hepatocellular carcinoma results from chronic cyclin D1 overexpression in transgenic mice. Cancer Res 61:5389–5395

22. Spataro V, Norbury C, Harris AL (1998) The ubiquitin-proteasome pathway in cancer. Br J Cancer 77:448–455

23. Bartek J, Lukas J (2001) Cell cycle. Order from destruction. Science 294:66–67

24. Lara-Pezzi E, Majano PL, Gomez-Gonzalo M, Garcia-Monzon C, Moreno-Otero R, Levrero M, Lopez-Cabrera M (1998) The hepatitis B virus X protein up-regulates tumor necrosis factor alpha gene expression in hepatocytes. Hepatology 28:1013–1021

Subject Index

If you have any concerns about our products,
you can contact us on
ProductSafety@springernature.com

In case Publisher is established outside the EU,
the EU authorized representative is:
Springer Nature Customer Service Center GmbH
Europaplatz 3, 69115 Heidelberg, Germany

Printed by Libri Plureos GmbH
in Hamburg, Germany